Real Superfoods Diet Cookbook

Nourishing the Natural Way, 120+ Healthy and Delicious Recipes for Lifelong Wellness

Valerie R. Johnson

Copyright page

All right reserved, no part of this publication may be republished in any form or by any means, including photocopy, scanning or otherwise without prior written permission to the copyright holder.

Table of Content

Introduction

Introducing the culinary adventure that promises to revolutionize not only your eating habits but also your overall lifestyle - the "Real Superfoods Diet Cookbook: Nourishing the Natural Way." These pages are a symphony of flavors that combine nutritional acumen with culinary mastery to reinvent the essence of a healthy lifestyle and improve your overall well-being.

This cookbook is a light of honesty in a world full of fads and diet trends, pointing you in the direction of a fulfilling and sustainable path. Written by the master chef Valerie R. Johnson, this compilation of more than 120 recipes is more than simply a recipe book—it's a starting point for a journey toward perpetual well-being.

Get ready to go on a taste journey that takes you beyond the ordinary and into a world where pleasure and health coexist together. These dishes are a fine blend of flavor and wellness, carefully selected to please your palette and nourish your body, rather than just satisfying dietary requirements.

The "Real Superfoods Diet Cookbook" is a celebration of bright health and vigor rather than a manifesto for dieting. It reveals the remarkable influence superfoods—nature's nutritional jewels— have on your general health and wellbeing. Here, food serves as more than simply nourishment; it is an essential tool for creating a long, vibrant life.

What Is Unique About This Cookbook?

- **The Merge of Nutritional Science and Culinary Art:**

Every recipe is a work of culinary art that combines nutritional science with artistic sensibility. Every element, from the creative presentation to the choice of ingredients, demonstrates the author's dedication to quality.

- **120+ Personalized Recipes:**

Both your travel and your dietary requirements are distinct. This cookbook, with more than 120 dishes, accommodates a wide range of dietary requirements, tastes, and wellness objectives. There's a recipe designed specifically for you, no matter how experienced you are in the kitchen.

- **A Superfood Symphony:**

Take in the symphony of superfoods, which are antioxidant- and nutrient-rich components that serve as the basis for every cuisine. Discover the culinary magic of foods praised for their ability to improve health, from quinoa to kale, berries to avocados.

- **Pleasure Meets Pragmatism:**

These recipes, which acknowledge the realities of contemporary life, skillfully combine use and enjoyment. Time constraints and rigorous schedules are no longer barriers; rather, they present chances to enjoy nutritious, tasty, and fast meals.

Take this cookbook as an invitation to go on a lifetime wellness adventure as you flip through the pages. One recipe at a time, each leading to a brighter, healthier self. Savor the joys of healthful foods, embrace the joy of intentionally feeding your body, and enjoy the exquisite tastes that are in store for you.

Prepare to go off on a gourmet adventure beyond the ordinary, where health becomes a way of life rather than a destination. Greetings from the "Real Superfoods Diet Cookbook," where each dish is an ode to your well-being and an evidence of the remarkable joy that comes from feeding your body naturally.

Chapter 1

Understanding Superfoods: Definition and Criteria for Superfoods

Definition

Superfoods are nutrient-dense meals with a high concentration of vitamins, minerals, antioxidants, and other vital components that provide remarkable health advantages.

Criteria for Superfoods

Density of Nutrients: Superfoods have a high concentration of vital nutrients compared to their calorie content.

Antioxidant Content: Strong antioxidants found in them help to prevent oxidative stress and support general health.

Health advantages: There are a number of health advantages linked to superfoods, including better heart health and increased cognitive performance.

Importance of Superfoods in Achieving Optimal Health

Superfoods provide the body with a wide variety of important nutrients that are necessary for general health and vigor, making them nutritional powerhouses.

Disease Prevention: Studies have shown that regular consumption of superfoods lowers the chance of developing chronic illnesses including diabetes, cardiovascular problems, and some forms of cancer.

Energy and vigor: The nutritional makeup of superfoods supports both physical and mental vigor throughout the day by sustaining high levels of energy.

Anti-Inflammatory Properties: A lot of superfoods include anti-inflammatory qualities that aid the body in reducing inflammation, which is linked to a number of health problems.

Enhanced Cognitive Function: A decreased risk of age-related cognitive decline and an association with enhanced cognitive function have been linked to specific superfoods, such blueberries and fatty salmon.

Guide to Incorporating Superfoods into Daily Meals

For a supercharged start to your morning smoothie or oatmeal, add spinach, chia seeds, or berries.

Superfood Swaps: Use superfoods to replace common items in recipes. For example, use quinoa in lieu of rice or add kale to salads.

Snack Wisely: To provide yourself with a filling and healthy lunchtime boost, choose for superfood snacks such as nuts, seeds, or Greek yogurt with honey.

<u>Vibrant Plate Technique:</u>

Include a range of fruits and vegetables on your plate to achieve a colorful dish, since each one offers a distinct set of nutrients.

Add Whole Grains: To increase the amount of fiber and nutrients in meals, choose whole grains such brown rice, quinoa, or farro.

Herbs and Spices: Take use of the therapeutic and anti-inflammatory qualities of herbs and spices such as garlic, ginger, and turmeric.

Meal Prep with Superfoods: To make eating easier, batch-cook meals with superfoods, such as sweet potatoes, legumes, and leafy greens.

Superfood-infused water is delicious and a great way to stay hydrated. Try infusing water with pieces of citrus fruit, cucumber, or mint.

A revolutionary step in attaining maximum health is comprehending and implementing superfoods into regular meals. People may take advantage of the remarkable health advantages that superfoods provide by adopting nutrient-rich choices and incorporating them into a varied and well-balanced diet. This all-encompassing method not only improves physical health but also supports a lively and active way of living.

Chapter 2:

Breakfasts for a Powerful Start

<u>Almond and Blueberry Pancakes</u>

Description: A tasty and gluten-free breakfast alternative, these fluffy pancakes made with almond flour and blueberries are topped with a drizzle of pure maple syrup.

Prep time: 15 minutes

Cooking time: 10 minutes

Number of Pancakes per Serving: 2–3

Ingredients:

- 1 cup almond flour;
- 1 teaspoon baking powder;

Preparation Guide:

1. In a bowl, thoroughly mix almond flour, baking powder, eggs, and almond milk.
2. Add 1/2 cup almond milk.
3. Add a handful of blueberries.
4. Drizzle with pure maple syrup.
5. Cook spoonful of batter on a hot, greased griddle after folding in the blueberries.
6. Garnish with a dollop of real maple syrup.

Legumes Mediterranean

Description: A flavorful and portable breakfast of protein-rich egg muffins flavored with Mediterranean herbs and topped with cherry tomatoes, feta cheese, and olives.

Prep time: 10 minutes

Cooking time: 20 minutes

Two muffins per serving

Ingredients

- 4 eggs, halved cherry tomatoes
- crumbled Feta cheese
- sliced olives
- chopped fresh basil

Preparation Guide

1. After whisking the eggs, fill the muffin cups.

2. Fill each cup with cherry tomatoes, feta, olives, and fresh basil.

3. Bake for the savory Mediterranean egg muffins until the eggs are set.

Omelette with Spinach and Feta Cheese

Description: A savory dish that combines cherry tomatoes, feta cheese, and fresh spinach for a filling and protein-rich breakfast.

Prep time: 10 minutes

Cooking time: 5 minutes

1 serving

Ingredients:

- Handful of fresh spinach
- cup crumbled feta cheese
- cup halved cherry tomatoes
- Season with salt and pepper to taste

Preparation Guide:

1. Beat eggs and transfer to a hot, well-oiled pan.
2. Fill one side of the omelette with spinach, feta, and tomatoes.
3. After folding, cook the omelette until the eggs are set.

Green Smoothie Bowl

Description: A nutrient-dense smoothie bowl with spinach, banana, and pineapple is garnished with chia seeds, coconut flakes, and granola for a filling and refreshing breakfast.

Prep time: 5 Minutes

Cooking time: 0-1 minutes

1 Serving

Ingredients

- 1/2 cup almond milk;

- 1/2 cup pineapple chunks
- For the topping, combine granola, coconut flakes, and chia seeds.

Preparation Guide:

1. Blend spinach, banana, pineapple, and almond milk until smooth.

2. Transfer to a bowl and garnish with chia seeds, coconut flakes, and granola.

<u>Revitalizing Acai Bowl</u>

Description: A colorful and antioxidant-packed bowl made with blended banana and acai berries, garnished with fresh berries, granola, and honey.

Prep time: 10 Minutes

1 Serving

Ingredients:

- One package of frozen acai puree, one banana
- 1/2 cup almond milk; 1/2 cup granola; fresh berries for garnish; and a drizzle of honey

Preparation Guide

1. Blend almond milk, banana, and acai puree until smooth.

2. Transfer to a bowl and garnish with fresh berries, granola, and honey.

Quinoa and Berry Breakfast dish

Description: A high-protein dish made with cooked quinoa, Greek yogurt, and a mixture of fresh berries, along with a dash of chia seeds, is presented.

Prep time: 15 minutes

Cooking time: 15 minutes

1 Serving size

Ingredients:

- half a cup cooked quinoa and half a cup Greek yogurt
- One tablespoon of chia seeds
- Mixed berries (strawberries, blueberries, and raspberries)
- Optional maple syrup drizzle

Preparation Guide:

1. Combine Greek yogurt and cooked quinoa.
2. If preferred, garnish with chia seeds, mixed berries, and a drizzle of maple syrup.

Chia Seed Pudding Parfait

Description: A tasty parfait that combines chia seeds, Greek yogurt, and sliced kiwi to create a visually pleasing and healthful dish.

Prep time: 5 minutes (including chilling time for the chia pudding)

1 serving

Ingredients:

- 2 teaspoons chia seeds
- 1/2 cup almond milk,
- 1/2 cup Greek yogurt.
- Top with sliced kiwis
- Garnish with optional agave syrup

Preparation Guide:

1. Combine chia seeds and almond milk; refrigerate until thickened, generally several hours or overnight.
2. Arrange Greek yogurt and chia pudding in a glass.
3. Place sliced kiwis on top, and if like, sprinkle with agave syrup.

Breakfast tortilla with Sweet Potatoes and Black Beans

Description: A filling tortilla that combines roasted sweet potatoes, black beans, scrambled eggs, and avocado, providing a delightful combination of tastes and textures.

Prep time: 15 minutes

Cooking time: 20 minutes

1 Serving

Ingredients:

- 1 whole-grain tortilla
- 1/2 cup diced roasted sweet potatoes
- 1/4 cup cooked black beans; and 2 scrambled eggs.
- Topping: sliced avocado and salad;

Preparation Guide:

- Stuff the tortilla with scrambled eggs, black beans, and roasted sweet potatoes.
- Add sliced avocado and salsa on top.

Banana and Almond Butter Overnight Oats

Description: Rolling oats are soaked in almond milk for a fast and healthy overnight oats meal. Almond butter, banana slices, and a dash of cinnamon are added on top.

Prep Time: 5 minutes (including oats chilling time)

Cooking Time: 0-1 minutes;

1 **Serving**

Ingredients:

pg. 17

- 1/2 cup rolled oats
- 1/2 cup almond milk
- 1 tablespoon almond butter
- 1 sliced banana
- One pinch of cinnamon

Preparation Guide:

1. Whisk together rolled oats and almond milk, then refrigerate overnight.
2. Before serving, top with banana slices, almond butter, and a dash of cinnamon.

Avocado and Smoked Salmon bread

Description: A classy yet straightforward breakfast consisting of smoked salmon and mashed avocado over whole-grain bread, topped with fresh dill and lemon zest.

Prep time: 10 minutes

Cooking time: is 0-1 minutes

1 **Serving**

Ingredients

- Smoked salmon slices,
- mashed avocado,
- toasted whole-grain bread,
- Lemon zest, and fresh dill for garnish.

Preparation Guide:

1. Spread the mashed avocado on the toasted bread.
2. Cover with smoked salmon and sprinkle with fresh dill and lemon zest.

These breakfast dishes combine a range of tastes and textures with nutrient-dense foods to provide a satisfying start to your day. These dishes, which range from colorful smoothie bowls to flavorful egg muffins, satisfy a wide range of palates and dietary requirements while guaranteeing a satisfying and nutritious breakfast. Savor the potent advantages of a nutritious breakfast!

Energizing Smoothie Bowls

<u>Berry Bliss Smoothie Bowl</u>

Description: A cool, antioxidant-rich bowl with a mixture of mixed berries, banana, and Greek yogurt; granola and chia seeds are added on top.

Prep time: 5 minutes

Cooking time: 0-1 minutes.

Ingredients:

- 1 cup mixed berries (strawberries, blueberries, raspberries);
- 1 banana;
- Half a cup of yogurt
- Topping of granola with chia seeds

Preparation Guide:

1. Blend banana, Greek yogurt, and mixed berries until smooth.

2. Transfer to a bowl, then garnish with chia seeds and granola.

Tropical Paradise Smoothie Bowl

Description: A tropical flavor infused with a mixture of pineapple, mango, and coconut milk, finished with shredded coconut, sliced kiwi, and honey.

One serving size, five minutes of prep, zero minutes of cooking, and the following

Ingredients:

- One cup of chunk pineapple and half a cup of chunk mango.
- A half-cup of coconut milk
- Topping ingredients include sliced kiwi, shredded coconut, and honey.

Preparation Guide:

1. Blend pineapple, mango, and coconut milk until smooth.
2. Transfer to a bowl, then garnish with shredded coconut, sliced kiwis, and honey.

<u>Smoothie Bowl with Green Goddess Spinach</u>

Description: A very nutrient-dense dish of spinach, banana, and almond butter with sliced almonds, fresh berries, and hemp seeds on top.

Prep time; 5 minutes

Cooking time: 0-1 Minutes

1 serving size

Ingredients:

- 1 banana; 1 handful of fresh spinach
- One tsp almond butter
- Topped with hemp seeds, chopped almonds, and fresh berries;

Preparation Guide:

1. Blend spinach, banana, and almond butter until smooth.
2. Transfer to a bowl, then garnish with hemp seeds, fresh berries, and sliced almonds.

<u>Chocolate Peanut Butter Protein Bowl</u>

Description: A decadent and protein-rich bowl with peanut butter, banana, and chocolate protein powder, finished with granola and cocoa nibs.

Prep time: 5 minutes

Cooking time: 0-1 minutes

1 Serving

Ingredients:

- One scoop of chocolate protein powder
- one banana and two tablespoons of peanut butter
- Cacao nibs and granola as garnish

Preparation Guide:

1. Blend peanut butter, banana, and chocolate protein powder until smooth.
2. Transfer to a bowl and garnish with cacao nibs and granola.

Sunrise Citrus Smoothie Bowl

Description: A citrus-infused bowl with Greek yogurt, oranges, and mango combined with pomegranate seeds, citrus segments, and agave syrup drizzled on top.

Prep time: 5 minutes

Cooking time: 0-1 minutes

1 Serving

Ingredients:

- 1 orange, peeled and cut into segments
- 1/2 cup chopped mango
- 1/2 cup Greek yogurt
- Toppings of citrus segments, pomegranate seeds, and agave syrup

Preparation Guide:

1. Puree the mango, orange segments, and Greek yogurt until smooth.

2. Transfer to a bowl, then garnish with pomegranate seeds, citrus segments, and agave syrup.

Mocha Almond Smoothie Bowl

Description: The dish consists of almond milk, banana, coffee, and a trace of cocoa powder. It is garnished with almond slices, banana slices, and cocoa powder.

Prep time: 5 minutes

Cooking time: 0-1 minutes

1 Serving

Ingredients:

- 1 banana;
- 1 cup almond milk
- One tablespoon powdered cocoa

Preparation Guide:

- Almond milk, banana, and cocoa powder should be blended until smooth.
- Top with sliced almonds, banana slices, and chocolate powder.
- Transfer to a bowl, then garnish with almond slices, banana slices, and a dash of cocoa powder.

Pina Colada Smoothie Bowl

Description: A tropical haven consisting of a mixture of pineapple, coconut milk, and banana, finished with sliced kiwi, coconut flakes, and honey drizzle.

Prep time: 5 minutes

Cooking time: 0-1 minutes

1 Serving

Ingredients:

- 1 cup pineapple chunks,
- 1/2 cup coconut milk, and 1 banana.
- Topping ingredients: sliced kiwi, honey, and coconut flakes.

Preparation Guide:

1. Blend banana, coconut milk, and pineapple until smooth.
2. Transfer to a bowl and garnish with sliced kiwi, coconut flakes, and honey.

Detox Green Tea Smoothie Bowl

Description: Garnish with kiwis, chia seeds, and a drizzle of lemon juice, this bowl is a delicious and detoxifying combination of green tea, cucumber, and mint.

Prep time: 5 minutes

Cooking time: 0-1 minutes

1 Serving

Ingredients:

- 1 cup cooled green tea;
- 1/2 sliced and peeled cucumber;
- fresh mint leaves;
- kiwi, chia seeds, and lemon juice for garnish

Preparation Guide:

1. Until smooth, blend together mint, cucumber, and green tea.
2. Transfer to a bowl, then garnish with chia seeds, kiwis, and a squeeze of lemon juice.

Almond Joy Smoothie Bowl

Description: A chocolaty and nutty bowl with banana, coconut flakes, almond milk, and a touch of cacao powder, garnished with sliced coconut and almonds.

Prep time: 5 minutes

Cooking time: 0-1 minutes

1 Serving

Ingredients:

- One cup almond milk,
- half a cup coconut flakes, and one banana
- One tablespoon powdered cacao
- Almond slices and extra coconut flakes for garnish

Preparation Guide:

1. Process the banana, cacao powder, coconut flakes, and almond milk until smooth.

2. Transfer to a bowl and garnish with more coconut flakes and sliced almonds.

Very Berry Citrus Blast Bowl

Description: A riot of tastes with a fusion of mixed berries, citrus fruits, and orange juice, finished with a scattering of flaxseeds and fresh berries and citrus slices.

This recipe calls for the following

Ingredients:

- 1 cup mixed berries (strawberries, blueberries, raspberries);
- 1/2 cup orange juice; peel and segment citrus fruits (grapefruit, orange);
- And 5 minutes of prep time.
- Topping ingredients: fresh berries, citrus slices, and flaxseeds;

Preparation Guide:

1. Process orange juice, mixed berries, and citrus fruits in a blender until smooth.

2. Transfer to a bowl and garnish with flaxseeds, citrus slices, and fresh berries.

These recipes for energy-boosting smoothie bowls provide a delicious blend of tastes, textures, and nutrients. These bowls are made to provide you a boost of energy and sustenance to start your day, whether you're craving a tropical getaway, a high-protein treat, or a cooling detox. Savor the colorful and healthful deliciousness of these mouthwatering smoothie bowls!

Superfood-Packed Overnight Oats

Overnight Oats with Blueberry Bliss

Description: For a superfood-rich morning treat, try this delicious combination of oats, almond milk, and blueberries that have been soaked overnight.

Prep time: 5 minutes

1 Serving

Ingredients:

- Oats, half a cup rolled
- half a cup of almond milk
- a small handful of raw blueberries
- dripping honey

Preparation Guide:

1. In a container, combine almond milk and rolled oats.
2. Give the fresh blueberries a good toss.
3. Before serving, sprinkle some honey over the top and refrigerate for the entire night.

Almond Butter Crunch with Chia

Description: Classic overnight oats are elevated with creamy almond butter and nutrient-rich chia seeds to create a filling meal that may be garnished with sliced almonds for extra crunch.

Prep time: 5 minutes

1 Serving

Ingredients:

- Oats, half a cup rolled
- half a cup of almond milk
- One tsp almond butter
- One-third cup chia seeds
- Almond slices as a garnish

Preparation Guide:

1. In a container, mix rolled oats, almond butter, almond milk, and chia seeds.
2. When ready to serve, stir thoroughly, cover with sliced almonds, and chill overnight.

Green Goddess Matcha Oatmeal

Description: Harness the power of matcha's antioxidants to transform your morning. Almond milk and matcha powder are combined to create these overnight oats, which are then garnished with fresh strawberries and chia seeds.

Prep time: 5 minutes

1 Serving

Ingredients:

- Oats, half a cup rolled
- half a cup of almond milk
- One teaspoon powdered matcha
- Sliced Chia seeds and fresh strawberries as a topping

Preparation Guide:

1. In a container, combine matcha powder, almond milk, and rolled oats.
2. Before serving, cover with chia seeds and fresh strawberries and refrigerate overnight.

Power Bowl with Peanut Butter and Bananas

Description: A protein-rich treat with the traditional peanut butter and banana combination. A substantial foundation for this superfood-filled overnight oats dish is provided by rolled oats and chia seeds.

Prep time: 5 minutes

1 Serving

Ingredients:

- Oats, half a cup rolled
- half a cup of almond milk
- One tsp peanut butter
- One banana, cut.

Preparation Guide:

1. In a container, mix peanut butter, almond milk, and rolled oats.

2. Serve after thoroughly stirring, chilling for the entire night, and garnish with sliced bananas.

Paradise of Coconut and Mango

Description: These overnight oats laced with coconut and mango will take you to a tropical paradise. A vacation in a jar, garnished with shredded coconut and juicy mango chunks.

Prep time: 5 minutes

1 Serving

Ingredients:

- Oats, half a cup rolled
- half a cup of coconut milk
- Mango slices fresh
- Add shredded coconut as a garnish.

Preparation Guide:

1. In a container, combine coconut milk and rolled oats.
2. Before serving, garnish with shredded coconut and fresh mango pieces after refrigerated for the entire night.

The Overnight Delight of Cacao Crunch

Description: Savor the deep aromas of chocolate with these overnight oats flavored with cacao. topped with sliced bananas and, for an added crunch, a dusting of cocoa nibs.

Prep time: 5 minutes

1 Serving

Ingredients:

- Oats, half a cup rolled
- half a cup of almond milk
- One tablespoon powdered cacao
- Slices of banana
- Cocoa nibs as a garnish

Preparation Guide:

1. In a container, mix almond milk, cacao powder, and rolled oats.
2. Before serving, garnish with banana slices and cacao nibs after refrigerated for the entire night.

Elegance of Pomegranates and Pistachios

Description: Add some elegance and crunch to your morning ritual with pomegranate and pistachio. The tastes and textures in these overnight oats are harmonious.

Prep time: 5 minutes

1 Serving

Ingredients:

- Oats, half a cup rolled
- half a cup of almond milk
- Young pomegranate seeds
- Add pistachios on top.

Preparation Guide:

1. In a container, combine almond milk and rolled oats.
2. Before serving, garnish with freshly chopped pistachios and pomegranate arils and refrigerate overnight.

Golden Bowl with Turmeric and Ginger

Description: Use the anti-inflammatory properties of ginger and turmeric in this recipe for golden-hued overnight oats. Finished with sliced kiwis and a honey drizzle for extra sweetness.

Prep time: 5 minutes

1 Serving

Ingredients:

- Oats, half a cup rolled
- half a cup of coconut milk
- one-half tsp turmeric powder
- half a tsp finely grated ginger
- Kiwi slices with honey as a garnish

Preparation Guide:

1. In a container, mix rolled oats, coconut milk, grated ginger, and turmeric powder.
2. Before serving, garnish with sliced kiwis and a honey drizzle after refrigerated for the entire night.

Superfood Delight: Apple Cinnamon Apple

Description: Indulge in the time-tested pairing of apple and cinnamon with these nutrient-dense overnight oats. For a cozy breakfast, add some cinnamon and apple slices over top.

Prep time: 5 minutes

1 Serving

Ingredients:

1. Oats, half a cup rolled
2. half a cup of almond milk
3. sliced apples
4. pulverized cinnamon for garnish

Preparation Guide:

1. In a container, combine almond milk and rolled oats.
2. Before serving, garnish with apple slices and a dusting of ground cinnamon after refrigerating for the whole night.

Power Bowl of Acai Berries

Description: Savor the benefits of acai berries, which are rich in antioxidants, with these overnight oats. Topped with a mixture of fresh berries and a delicious drizzle of agave syrup.

Prep time: 5 minutes

1 Serving

Ingredients:

1. Oats, half a cup rolled
2. half a cup of almond milk
3. Pureed acai berries (fresh or frozen)
4. Strawberries to decorate with and agave syrup to pour over

Preparation Guide:

1. In a container, mix rolled oats, almond milk, and pureed acai berries.
2. Before serving, garnish with a mixture of berries and a drizzle of agave syrup and refrigerate overnight.

These nutrient-dense overnight oats dishes are a tasty and easy way to start your day. They contain superfoods. There's a flavor-packed alternative for any morning taste, whether you're craving the pleasure of chocolate, the antioxidant benefits of berries, or the tropical vibes of coconut and mango. Savor the filling, nutritious goodness of these healthy overnight oats!

Nutrient-Dense Breakfast Muffins and Bites

Breakfast Muffins with Spinach and Feta

Description: A delicious and portable breakfast choice, these nutrient-packed muffins feature fresh spinach, feta cheese, and cherry tomatoes.

Size of Serving: 6 Muffins

Preparation Time: 20 minutes

Ingredients:

- Two cups chopped fresh spinach,
- one-half cup crumbled feta cheese,
- one-half cup cherry tomatoes, and six diced eggs
- Add pepper and salt to taste.

Preparation Guide:

1. Set a muffin tray to 350°F (175°C) and preheat the oven.
2. Whisk together the eggs in a bowl and mix in the diced cherry tomatoes, feta, and chopped spinach.
3. Add pepper and salt for seasoning.

4. Once the eggs have set, pour the mixture into the muffin tray and bake for 20 minutes.

Breakfast Bites of Banana and Walnut

Brief Description: A hearty and filling morning delight, these nutrient-dense pieces are made with chopped walnuts, oats, and ripe bananas.

Meal Size: Twelve Bits

Preparation Time: 15 minutes

Ingredients:

- two ripe, mashed bananas
- Oats, rolled, one cup
- chop half a cup of walnuts
- 1/4 cup of honey.
- One tsp vanilla essence

Preparation Guide:

1. Adjust the oven temperature to 350°F (175°C) and place parchment paper on a baking pan.
2. Combine mashed bananas, chopped walnuts, rolled oats, honey, and vanilla essence in a bowl.
3. Place parts on the baking sheet that are the size of tablespoons, and bake for 15 minutes, or until golden brown.

Quinoa and Sweet Potato Breakfast Muffins

Description: For a nutrient-dense and delectable breakfast, try these protein-rich muffins with cooked quinoa, sweet potatoes, and a touch of cinnamon.

Size of Serving: 8 Muffins

Preparation Time: 25 minutes

Ingredients:

- One cup of mashed sweet potatoes
- 1 cup of quinoa,
- cooked two eggs
- 1/4 of a cup maple syrup
- One tsp of cinnamon

Preparation Guide:

1. Set a muffin tray to 375°F (190°C) and preheat the oven.
2. Mashed sweet potatoes, cooked quinoa, eggs, cinnamon, and maple syrup should all be combined in a dish.
3. After filling the muffin tray, bake for 25 minutes, or until a toothpick inserted into the center comes out clean.

Almond-Blueberry Breakfast Bites

Description: A tasty and practical breakfast snack, these nutrient-dense pieces are overflowing with blueberries, almonds, and chia seeds.

Meal Size: Twelve Bits

Preparation Time: 20 minutes

Ingredients:

- One cup of berries
- half a cup of chopped almonds
- Half a cup of chia seeds
- Two tsp of honey
- One tsp almond extract

Preparation Guide:

1. Adjust the oven temperature to 350°F (175°C) and place parchment paper on a baking pan.
2. Blueberries, chopped almonds, chia seeds, honey, and almond essence should all be combined in a bowl.
3. Pour mixture onto baking sheet; bake until sides are golden brown, about 20 minutes.

Breakfast Muffins with Cheese and Veggies

Description: Savory and nourishing breakfast option: veggie-packed muffins stuffed with cheese, onions, and bell peppers.

Size of Serving: 6 Muffins

Preparation Time: 25 minutes

Ingredients:

- one-half cup chopped bell peppers
- Diced 1/4 cup red onion
- Six eggs, half a cup of shredded cheddar cheese
- Add pepper and salt to taste.

Preparation Guide:

1. Set a muffin tray to 375°F (190°C) and preheat the oven.
2. Whisk eggs in a basin and add shredded cheddar cheese, chopped bell peppers, and red onion.
3. Add pepper and salt for seasoning.
4. Once the eggs are set, pour the mixture into the muffin tray and bake for 25 minutes.

Breakfast Bites with Apple and Cinnamon

Description: Packed with of nutrients, these bite-sized treats with chopped apples, oats, and a hint of cinnamon provide a tasty and healthy breakfast option.

Meal Size: Twelve Bits

Preparation Time: 20 minutes

Ingredients:

1. one cup of diced apples
2. Oats, rolled, one cup
3. one-fourth cup almond butter
4. Two tsp pure maple syrup
5. One tsp of cinnamon

Preparation Guide:

1. Adjust the oven temperature to 350°F (175°C) and place parchment paper on a baking pan.
2. Combine rolled oats, almond butter, cinnamon, maple syrup, and chopped apples in a bowl.
3. Place sections on the baking sheet, about the size of a tablespoon, and bake for 20 minutes, or until the edges are golden brown.

Southwestern-Style Egg Muffins

Description: A savory and Mediterranean-inspired breakfast alternative, these protein-rich muffins are topped with cherry tomatoes, feta cheese, and olives.

Size of Serving: 6 Muffins

Preparation Time: 20 minutes

Ingredients:

- half a cup of chopped cherry tomatoes
- 1/4 cup of crumbled feta cheese
- 1/4 cup chopped Kalamata olives with 6 eggs
- Add pepper and salt to taste.

Preparation Guide:

1. Set a muffin tray to 375°F (190°C) and preheat the oven.
2. Whisk together the eggs in a bowl and mix in the feta cheese, chopped olives, and diced cherry tomatoes. Add pepper and salt for seasoning.
3. Once the eggs have set, pour the mixture into the muffin tray and bake for 20 minutes.

Breakfast Muffins with Chocolate Zucchini

Description: These nutrient-dense muffins with shredded zucchini and cocoa powder are a tasty and cunning way to eat vegetables for breakfast.

Size of Serving: 8 Muffins

Preparation Time: 25 minutes

Ingredients:

- One cup of shredded and drained zucchini
- 1/4 cup powdered cocoa
- Two eggs and 1/4 cup honey
- One tsp vanilla essence

Preparation Guide:

1. Set a muffin tray to 350°F (175°C) and preheat the oven.
2. Shredded zucchini, eggs, honey, cocoa powder, and vanilla essence should all be combined in a bowl.
3. After filling the muffin tray, bake for 25 minutes, or until a toothpick inserted into the center comes out clean.

<u>Oatmeal with Blueberries and Oats</u>

Description: Almond butter, oats, and blueberries combine to create nutrient-dense bits that make a filling and healthy morning treat.

Meal Size: Twelve Bits

Preparation Time: 20 minutes

Ingredients:

- One cup of berries
- Oats, rolled, one cup
- one-fourth cup almond butter
- Two tsp of honey
- One tsp vanilla essence

Preparation Guide:

1. Adjust the oven temperature to 350°F (175°C) and place parchment paper on a baking pan.
2. Blueberries, rolled oats, almond butter, honey, and vanilla essence should all be combined in a bowl.
3. Place sections on the baking sheet, about the size of a tablespoon, and bake for 20 minutes, or until the edges are golden brown.

Breakfast Muffins with Cheddar and Broccoli

Description: Savory and nutrient-dense breakfast option—vegetable-packed muffins with cheddar cheese and broccoli.

Size of Serving: 6 Muffins

Preparation Time: 25 minutes

Ingredients:

- Half a cup of finely chopped broccoli
- Six eggs, half a cup of shredded cheddar cheese
- Add pepper and salt to taste.

Preparation Guide:

1. Set a muffin tray to 375°F (190°C) and preheat the oven.
2. Whisk together the eggs in a basin and mix in the shredded cheddar cheese and finely chopped broccoli.
3. Add pepper and salt for seasoning.
4. Once the eggs are set, pour the mixture into the muffin tray and bake for 25 minutes.

From savory to sweet, these nutrient-dense breakfast muffins and bites provide a range of tastes and ingredients, making them a simple and healthy addition to your daily routine. Savor the deliciousness of these filling and tasty breakfast foods!

Chapter 3

Lunches for Sustained Energy

<u>Quinoa Salad with Tahini-Lemon Dressing</u>

Description: A colorful quinoa salad with chickpeas, fresh veggies, and a zesty lemon-tahini dressing that makes for a filling and energetic lunch.

Size of Serving: 2

15 minutes is the cooking time for quinoa.

Ingredients:

- One cup of cooked quinoa
- Mixed veggies, including bell peppers, cucumbers, and cherry tomatoes
- 1 can of drained chickpeas
- freshly cut parsley
- Salted and peppered, with 3 tablespoons of tahini, 2 teaspoons of lemon juice, and 1 tablespoon of olive oil for dressing

Preparation Guide:

1. Put the cooked quinoa, chickpeas, mixed veggies, and fresh parsley in a bowl.
2. To make the dressing, combine the tahini, lemon juice, olive oil, salt, and pepper in a another bowl.
3. After adding the dressing to the salad, gently mix to fully incorporate.

Bowl of Quinoa with Grilled Chicken

Description: For a filling and healthy lunch, try this protein-rich bowl of quinoa, roasted veggies, and grilled chicken drizzled with balsamic sauce.

One serving size

Preparation Time: 20 minutes

Ingredients:

- 1 chicken breast, skin and boneless
- Half a cup of cooked quinoa
- Roasted mixed veggies (bell peppers, cherry tomatoes, and zucchini)
- Marzipan glaze

Preparation Guide:

1. Cook the chicken breast on the grill until it's done.
2. Combine the grilled chicken, roasted veggies, and cooked quinoa in a bowl.
3. Before serving, drizzle with balsamic glaze.

Wrap with Mediterranean Chickpeas

Description: A wrap with a Mediterranean flair that is stuffed with fresh veggies, feta cheese, seasoned chickpeas, and a zesty tzatziki sauce.

15 minutes for preparation

Five minutes for cooking

2 Serving

Ingredients:

- One can of washed and drained chickpeas
- Various greens
- Cucumber cut in half, crumbled Feta cheese, cherry tomatoes
- Whole-wheat tortillas
- Sauce Tzatziki

Preparation Guide:

1. Heat up some chickpeas seasoned with your preferred spices in a skillet.
2. Put together wraps with feta cheese, cucumber, cherry tomatoes, sautéed chickpeas, mixed greens, and tzatziki sauce drizzled over.

Quinoa Bowl with Salmon and Avocado

Description: For a tasty and filling lunch, try this nutrient-rich dish of grilled salmon, avocado slices, quinoa, and zesty vinaigrette.

15 minutes for preparation

Ten minutes for cooking

2 Serving

Ingredients:

- 1 fillet of salmon
- Half a cup cooked quinoa with chopped avocado
- Various greens

- Two tablespoons olive oil, one tablespoon lemon juice, one teaspoon Dijon mustard, salt, and pepper make up the vinaigrette.

Preparation Guide:

1. You may cook the salmon fillet on the grill until it's done.
2. Put the cooked quinoa, avocado slices, and mixed greens in a bowl.
3. To make the vinaigrette, whisk together olive oil, lemon juice, Dijon mustard, salt, and pepper.
4. Place the grilled salmon on top of the bowl and pour the zesty vinaigrette over it.

Buddha Bowl with Sweet Potatoes and Black Beans

Description: A filling and well-balanced lunch dish consisting of quinoa, black beans, roasted sweet potatoes, and a cilantro-lime vinaigrette.

One serving size

Preparation Time: 25 minutes

Ingredients:

- One big sweet potato, cut into pieces and baked
- half a cup of cooked black beans
- Half a cup of cooked quinoa
- Various greens
- 3 tablespoons olive oil, 1 tablespoon lime juice, fresh cilantro, salt, and pepper are used to make the dressing.

Preparation Guide:

1. Sweet potatoes should be roasted in the oven until golden brown.
2. Black beans, quinoa, mixed greens, and roasted sweet potatoes should all be combined in a dish.
3. To make the dressing, blend together olive oil, lime juice, fresh cilantro, salt, and pepper. Over the Buddha bowl, drizzle.

Mango and Shrimp Salad

Description: A crisp salad that perfectly balances flavors and textures with grilled shrimp, juicy mango, avocado, and tangy vinaigrette.

Size of Serving: 2

Five minutes for cooking

Ingredients:

- 1/2 pound of deveined and peeled shrimp
- Diced avocado, sliced ripe mango
- Various greens
- Two tablespoons olive oil, one tablespoon orange juice, one teaspoon honey, salt, and pepper make up the vinaigrette.

Preparation Guide:

1. Turn shrimp over and heat until done.
2. Grilled shrimp, chopped mango, avocado slices, and mixed greens should all be combined in a dish.

3. To make the vinaigrette, whisk together olive oil, honey, orange juice, salt, and pepper. Pour over the greens.

Stir-fried Vegetables and Chicken with Asian Flavors

Description: For a well-balanced lunch, try this delectable and speedy stir-fried chicken with vibrant veggies and a savory sauce with Asian inspiration, all served over brown rice.

Size of Serving: 2

Preparation Time: 15 minutes

Ingredients:

- One pound of finely sliced, boneless, skinless chicken breast
- Sliced mixed veggies (broccoli, bell peppers, and snap peas)
- One cup cooked brown rice.
- Three tablespoons soy sauce, one oyster sauce tablespoon, one sesame oil tablespoon, and one teaspoon cornstarch make up the sauce.

Preparation Guide:

1. Cook and brown the chicken by stirring-frying it in a wok or pan.
2. Vegetables should be added and cooked until crisp-tender.
3. To make the sauce, combine the soy sauce, oyster sauce, sesame oil, and cornstarch in a small bowl.

4. After adding the sauce, mix the stir-fry until it is well covered. Place on top of warm brown rice.

<u>Vegetable and Lentil Stew</u>

Description: A filling and substantial meal, this stew is full of flavor and nutrients and contains lentils, a variety of veggies, and fragrant spices.

15 minutes for preparation

Cooking Period: Half an hour

4 Serving

Ingredients:

- One cup of washed and dried brown or green lentils
- diced mixed veggies (carrots, celery, and tomatoes)
- One onion, chopped finely
- three minced garlic cloves
- veggie-based soup
- Seasonings: paprika, cumin, coriander, salt, and pepper

Preparation Guide:

1. Add the garlic and onions to a large saucepan and sauté until softened.
2. Stir in spices, mixed veggies, and lentils. To coat, stir.
3. Add enough vegetable broth to the ingredients to cover them.
4. Cook until the veggies and lentils are soft. Taste and adjust seasoning.

Bowl of Caprese Quinoa

Description: A delicious quinoa bowl with fresh mozzarella, basil, cherry tomatoes, and balsamic sauce for a satisfyingly light lunch that pays homage to the traditional Caprese salad.

Size of Serving: 2

Prep time: 15 minutes.

Ingredients:

- One cup of cooked quinoa
- Half a cherry tomato
- new mozzarella sticks
- fresh leaves of basil
- Marzipan glaze

Preparation Guide:

1. Cooked quinoa, cherry tomatoes, fresh mozzarella balls, and fresh basil leaves should all be combined in a dish.
2. Before serving, drizzle with balsamic glaze.

Stir-fried Teriyaki Tofu with Veggies

Description: A tasty plant-based stir-fry with jasmine rice, colorful veggies, and tofu topped with a homemade teriyaki sauce.

Size of Serving: 2

Preparation Time: 15 minutes

Ingredients:

- 1 block diced and pressed firm tofu

- Sliced mixed veggies (carrots, bell peppers, and broccoli)
- One cup cooked jasmine rice
- 3 tablespoons soy sauce, 2 teaspoons mirin, 1 tablespoon brown sugar, 1 teaspoon grated ginger, and 1 chopped garlic clove make up the Teriyaki Sauce.

Preparation Guide:

1. Sauté cubed tofu in a wok or skillet until golden brown.
2. Vegetables should be added and cooked until crisp-tender.
3. To make the teriyaki sauce, combine the soy sauce, mirin, brown sugar, grated ginger, and chopped garlic in a small bowl.
4. After adding the sauce, mix the stir-fry until it is well covered. Over cooked jasmine rice, serve.

These lunch ideas combine a range of foods, tastes, and nutrients to deliver you continuous energy and satisfaction throughout the day. Whether you're in the mood for a robust stew, a colorful salad, or a zesty stir-fry, these dishes provide tasty and nutritious alternatives for your noon meal. Savor the harmony of flavor and nourishment!

Superfood Salads and Dressings

Lemon-Tahini Dressed Quinoa Power Salad

Description: A nutrient-dense salad with avocado, cherry tomatoes, kale, and quinoa that is topped with a zesty lemon-tahini dressing for a filling and invigorating dinner.

Size of Serving: 2

15 minutes for preparation

Ingredients:

- 1 cup of quinoa, cooked
- Two cups chopped kale, sliced cherry tomatoes, one avocado cut in half
- Dressing made of lemon juice, tahini, olive oil, and salt

Preparation Guide:

1. Diced avocado, cherry tomatoes, chopped kale, and cooked quinoa should all be combined in a big dish.
2. Combine the ingredients for the lemon-tahini dressing in a separate bowl.
3. After adding the dressing to the salad, stir to fully incorporate.

Ginger-Miso Dressed Rainbow Detox Salad

Description: A bright and refreshing detox salad with bell peppers, carrots, and purple cabbage mixed together and dressed with a zesty ginger-miso dressing.

20 minutes for preparation

Size of Serving: 4

Ingredients:

1. julienned purple cabbage,
2. Thinly sliced carrots, red, yellow, and orange bell peppers,
3. Shredded ginger-miso dressing (ginger, miso paste, rice vinegar, sesame oil, and honey).

Preparation Guide:

1. In a big bowl, mix shredded purple cabbage, julienned carrots, and bell pepper slices.
2. Mix the ingredients for the ginger-miso dressing in a separate bowl.
3. After drizzling the salad with dressing, toss to coat well.

Balsamic Vinaigrette Kale and Blueberry Superfood Salad

Description: A delicious combination of tastes, tangy balsamic vinaigrette drizzles over a nutrient-rich salad of kale, blueberries, walnuts, and feta cheese.

Size of Serving: 2

15 minutes for preparation

Ingredients:

- 4 cups chopped kale greens with the stems removed
- One cup of berries
- 1/2 cup chopped walnuts and 1/4 cup crumbled feta cheese
- Balsamic vinaigrette (olive oil, honey, Dijon mustard, and balsamic vinegar)

Preparation Guide:

1. Chopped kale, blueberries, chopped walnuts, and crumbled feta cheese should all be combined in a big salad dish.
2. Mix the ingredients for the balsamic vinaigrette in a small basin.

3. Over the salad, drizzle with the vinaigrette and toss lightly to mix.

Tzatziki Dressed Mediterranean Quinoa Salad with Greek Yogurt

Description: A quinoa salad with cucumber, cherry tomatoes, Kalamata olives, feta cheese, and a zesty Greek yogurt dressing, influenced by the Mediterranean cuisine.

Size of Serving: 4

20 minutes for preparation

Ingredients:

- 1 cup of quinoa, cooked
- Diced Cherry tomatoes, chopped Kalamata olives, sliced Feta cheese, cucumber, and crumbled Greek yogurt tzatziki sauce (made with cucumber, lemon juice, garlic, and dill)

Preparation Guide:

1. Cooked quinoa, chopped cucumber, cherry tomatoes, sliced Kalamata olives, and crumbled feta cheese should all be combined in a big dish.
2. Combine the ingredients for the Greek yogurt tzatziki dressing in a blender.
3. After adding the dressing to the salad, toss to evenly distribute it.

Legumes-Packed Chickpea Salad with Herb-Lemon Dressing

Description: A salad rich in protein that combines cucumber, cherry tomatoes, feta cheese, and chickpeas with a tangy vinaigrette of lemon and herbs.

Size of Serving: 3

15 minutes for preparation

Ingredients.

- Two cans of chickpeas,
- washed and drained cherry tomatoes,
- chopped Feta cheese, split cucumber,
- and crumbled lemon-herb vinaigrette (olive oil, fresh herbs, Dijon mustard) are the

Preparation Guide:

1. Chickpeas, sliced cucumber,
2. Cherry tomatoes, and crumbled feta cheese should all be combined in a large mixing dish.
3. Combine the ingredients for the lemon-herb vinaigrette in a small bowl.
4. Drizzle the salad with the vinaigrette and gently toss to coat.

Edamame Salad with Sesame-Ginger Dressing, Inspired by Asian Cuisine

Description: An Asian-style salad with bell peppers, red cabbage, shredded carrots, and edamame combined with a tasty sesame-ginger vinaigrette.

Size of Serving: 4

Prepare Duration: 15 minutes.

Ingredients:

- 2 cups edamame,
- Thinly sliced sesame-ginger dressing (soy sauce, sesame oil, rice vinegar, ginger, garlic),
- Steamed red cabbage, shredded carrots, and shredded bell peppers (red and yellow).

Preparation Guide:

1. Steamed edamame, shredded carrots, shredded red cabbage, and sliced bell peppers should all be combined in a big salad dish.
2. Mix the ingredients for the sesame-ginger dressing in a small bowl.
3. Over the salad, drizzle with the dressing and stir until thoroughly mixed.

Quinoa Bowl with Roasted Vegetables and Lemon-Tahini Dressing

Description: A filling bowl of quinoa topped with a delicious lemon-tahini sauce with roasted veggies including sweet potatoes, Brussels sprouts, and red onions.

Prepare Duration: 20 minutes.

Cooking time (for roasting): thirty minutes

Size of Serving: 3

Ingredients:

- 1 cup of quinoa, cooked
- Diced Brussels sprouts, sweet potatoes, half red onions,
- and sliced lemon-tahini dressing (olive oil, garlic, tahini, and lemon juice)

Preparation Guide:

1. Roast the sliced red onions, chopped sweet potatoes, and half Brussels sprouts in a preheated oven until they are soft and golden.
2. Combine the roasted veggies and cooked quinoa in a large bowl.
3. Pour the lemon-tahini dressing into the bowl, then give it a little toss to coat.

Strawberry-Spinach Salad with Balsamic-Honey Dressing

Description: A light salad with baby spinach, almonds, goat cheese, and sliced strawberries dressed with a delicious balsamic-honey vinaigrette.

Ten minutes to prepare.

Size of Serving: 2

Ingredients:

- Four cups baby kale
- cut strawberries
- Almond crumbles, sliced goat cheese
- Honey-balsamic vinaigrette (made with honey, olive oil, Dijon mustard, and balsamic vinegar)

Preparation Guide:

1. Combine baby spinach, almond slices, crumbled goat cheese, and strawberry slices in a large salad dish.
2. Combine the ingredients for the balsamic-honey vinaigrette in a small bowl.
3. Over the salad, drizzle with the vinaigrette and toss lightly to mix.

Fiesta Salad with Avocado and Black Beans with Lime-Cilantro Dressing

Description: A zesty lime-cilantro salad with avocado, black beans, corn, and cherry tomatoes that is reminiscent of a fiesta.

Size of Serving: 4

15 minutes for preparation

Ingredients:

- Two avocados, cut up
- One can of well cleaned and emptied black beans
- kernels of corn, frozen or fresh
- Half a cherry tomato
- Dressing made of lime juice, cilantro, olive oil, and garlic

Preparation Guide:

1. Add the chopped avocados, black beans, corn kernels, and cherry tomatoes to a large salad dish.
2. Combine the ingredients for the lime-cilantro dressing in a small bowl.
3. After drizzling the salad with the dressing, gently toss to coat.

Chickpea and Super Green Salad with Tahini-Turmeric Dressing

Description: A colorful and nutrient-dense salad with a blend of cucumber, pumpkin seeds, chickpeas, and super greens, topped with a golden turmeric-tahini sauce.

15 minutes for preparation

Size of Serving: 3

Ingredients:

- Super greens mixed together (kale, spinach, arugula)

- One can of washed and drained chickpeas
- Diced cucumber
- Pimientos, or pumpkin seeds
- Olive oil, lemon juice, tahini, and turmeric combined to make a dressing.

Preparation Guide:

1. Diced cucumber, pumpkin seeds, chickpeas, and mixed super greens should all be combined in a big salad dish.
2. Mix the ingredients for the turmeric-tahini dressing in a small dish.
3. Over the salad, drizzle with the dressing and toss lightly to mix.

These recipes for superfood salads provide a delicious blend of tastes, textures, and health benefits. These salads, which feature detoxifying greens and protein-rich chickpeas, are topped with delectable homemade dressings to make for a filling and nutritious supper. Savor the colorful and nourishing richness of these dressings and salads made with superfoods!

Quick and Nutritious Lunch Wraps

<u>Veggie Mediterranean Wrap</u>

Description: A whole-grain tortilla encases a filling of feta cheese, cucumbers, cherry tomatoes, olives, and hummus, all wrapped in a cool and healthy wrap.

One serving size

Ten minutes to prepare.

Ingredients:

- A single wholegrain tortilla
- Half a cup of hummus
- Cherry tomatoes and cucumber slices cut in half
- Crumbled Feta cheese, sliced Kalamata olives, and

Preparation Guide:

1. Drizzle the whole-grain tortilla with hummus.
2. Add cherry tomatoes, cucumber slices, feta cheese crumbles, and olives to the layer.
3. Using a toothpick, seal the tortilla after rolling it into a wrap.

Peanut Wrap with Thai Chicken

Description: A spicy peanut sauce, grilled chicken, shredded cabbage, and carrots are all rolled up in a delicious spinach tortilla wrap.

One serving size

15 minutes for preparation

Ingredients:

- One tortilla with spinach
- Chicken strips grilled
- chopped cabbage
- Cut up carrots
- Peanut butter

Preparation Guide:

1. Flatten the tortilla with spinach.
2. Arrange the carrots, shredded cabbage, and grilled chicken.

3. Spread some peanut sauce over top, then fold it like a wrap.

Black bean and avocado wrap

Description: A filling whole-grain tortilla encases mashed avocado, black beans, corn, red onion, and cilantro, creating a delightful vegetarian wrap.

One serving size

Ten minutes to prepare.

Ingredients:

- A single wholegrain tortilla
- Mash one ripe avocado.
- Rinse and drain black beans
- Kernels of corn
- sliced red onion, finely
- chopped fresh cilantro

Preparation Guide:

1. Mashed avocado should be spread over the whole-grain tortilla.
2. Add fresh cilantro, red onion, corn, and black beans to the layer.
3. Cut in half after rolling into a wrap.

Chicken Caesar Wrap

Description: Grilled chicken, romaine lettuce, cherry tomatoes, parmesan cheese, and Caesar dressing combine to create a simple wrap version of the traditional Caesar salad.

One serving size

15 minutes for preparation

Ingredients:

- A single wholegrain tortilla
- Chicken strips grilled
- Romaine lettuce, shredded Caesar dressing, half a divided piece of Parmesan cheese, and sliced cherry tomatoes

Preparation Guide:

1. Spread out the whole-grain tortilla.
2. Arrange the cherry tomatoes, romaine lettuce, grilled chicken, and grated parmesan.
3. Spread over some Caesar dressing, then roll up and fold to form a wrap.

Veggie Caprese Wrap

Description: A sun-dried tomato tortilla encases a tasty and refreshing wrap with fresh mozzarella, tomatoes, basil, and balsamic sauce.

One serving size

Ten minutes to prepare.

Ingredients:

- One tortilla with sun-dried tomatoes
- Slabbed fresh mozzarella with sliced tomatoes
- fresh leaves of basil
- Marzipan glaze

Preparation Guide:

1. The sun-dried tomato tortilla should be placed on a level surface.
2. Arrange tomato slices, fresh mozzarella, and fresh basil in layers.
3. Spread some balsamic glaze over it and fold it up like a wrap.

<u>Veggie and Tofu Teriyaki Wrap</u>

Description: A tasty and filling wrap made with brown rice, stir-fried veggies, and tofu marinated in teriyaki sauce, all wrapped in a whole-grain tortilla.

One serving size

20 minutes for preparation

Ingredients:

- A single wholegrain tortilla
- Sliced tofu marinated in Teriyaki
- stir-fried veggies, such as carrots, broccoli, and bell peppers
- cooked brown rice

Preparation Guide:

1. Spread out the whole-grain tortilla.

2. Arrange the brown rice, stir-fried veggies, and pieces of teriyaki tofu.
3. Roll into a wrap and use toothpicks to secure if necessary.

Sun-Dried Tomato and Pesto Chicken Wrap

Description: A savory wrap made of spinach tortilla, grilled chicken, sun-dried tomatoes, pesto sauce, and feta cheese.

One serving size

15 minutes for preparation

Ingredients:

- One tortilla with spinach
- Chicken strips grilled
- Pesto pasta
- chopped sun-dried tomatoes
- fresh leaves of spinach
- Feta cheese, broken up

Preparation Guide:

1. Drizzle the spinach tortilla with pesto.
2. Add grilled chicken, crumbled feta, sun-dried tomatoes, and fresh spinach to the layer.
3. Cut in half after rolling into a wrap.

Chickpea and Buffalo Wrap

Description: A whole-grain tortilla encases a spicy and protein-rich wrap with chopped tomatoes, creamy avocado, shredded lettuce, and buffalo chickpeas.

One serving size

15 minutes for preparation

Ten minutes for cooking

Ingredient.

- One whole-grain tortilla is the Chickpeas from buffalo (cooked or canned)
- Tears from lettuce
- chopped tomato
- Sliced avocado

Preparation Guide:

1. Reheat the tortilla made of healthy grains.
2. Add sliced avocado, chopped tomatoes, shredded lettuce, and buffalo chickpeas to the layer.
3. Take a roll and savor it.

Roasted Vegetable Wrap with Hummus

Description: A filling whole-grain tortilla wrap stuffed with roasted veggies, hummus, and crumbled goat cheese. Ideal for vegetarians.

One serving size

20 minutes for preparation

Ingredients:

- A single wholegrain tortilla
- Roasted vegetables, such bell peppers, zucchini, and eggplant Hummus.
- Shreds of goat cheese

Preparation Guide:

1. Spread out the whole-grain tortilla.
2. Cover the tortilla with hummus.
3. Top with a heaping helping of goat cheese crumbles and roasted veggies.
4. Cut in half after rolling into a wrap.

<u>Cranberry and Turkey Wrap</u>

Description: A cranberry-walnut tortilla encases sliced turkey, stuffing, cranberry sauce, and a hint of cream cheese, creating a festive wrap.

One serving size

15 minutes for preparation

Ingredients:

- One walnut-cranberry tortilla
- Turkey slices with cranberry sauce
- Precooked stuffing
- Spread cheese

Preparation Guide:

1. Spread the walnut-cranberry tortilla out flat.

2. Arrange a layer of cream cheese, cranberry sauce, prepared stuffing, and turkey slices.

3. Enjoy after rolling into a festive wrap.

These easy and wholesome lunch wrap recipes come in a range of tastes and ingredients, which makes them ideal for a fulfilling midday meal. There's a tasty selection for every palate, ranging from teriyaki tofu and veggie wraps to Mediterranean vegetarian wraps. Savor these wraps as a healthy and convenient lunch option!

One-Pot Superfood Lunch Bowls

Power Bowl with Quinoa and Veggies

Description: A filling and healthy lunch dish made with quinoa, vibrant veggies, and a lemon-tahini sauce. Packed with nutrients.

Size of Serving: 2

Preparation Time: 20 minutes

Ingredients:

- One cup of washed quinoa
- Mixed veggies, including zucchini, cherry tomatoes, and bell peppers
- Cooked or canned chickpeas
- Tahini-lemon dressing

Preparation Guide:

1. Cook the mixed veggies and chickpeas in a saucepan until they become soft.

2. Add the cooked quinoa, chickpeas, and sautéed veggies together.
3. Pour in some lemon-tahini sauce.

Quinoa Bowl with Salmon and Broccoli

Description: A vibrant yogurt-dill sauce envelops quinoa, oven-roasted salmon, and steamed broccoli in a protein-rich dish.

Size of Serving: 2

Preparation Time: 25 minutes

Ingredients:

- One cup of washed quinoa
- Fish fillets
- Frolicking broccoli
- Greek yoghurt
- freshly sliced dill

Preparation Guide:

1. Broccoli should be steamed until soft, and fish should be baked.
2. Put broccoli, salmon, and quinoa in bowls.
3. Add some fresh dill and a dollop of Greek yogurt on top.

Chickpea and Spinach Bowl with Turmeric

Description: A colorful bowl of sautéed spinach, brown rice, and chickpeas flavored with turmeric, all topped with a creamy avocado-cilantro sauce.

Size of Serving: 2

Preparation Time: 20 minutes

Ingredients:

- One cup cooked brown rice
- Cooked or canned chickpeas
- new spinach
- For seasoning,
- Use paprika, cumin, and turmeric.
- cilantro-avocado sauce

Preparation Guide:

1. Follow the cooking directions on the package for brown rice.
2. Chickpeas should be sautéed till golden with paprika, cumin, and turmeric.
3. Wilt the fresh spinach in the same pan.
4. Put sautéed spinach, seasoned chickpeas, and brown rice into bowls. Drizzle with the cilantro-avocado sauce.

<u>Bowl of Mediterranean Quinoa Salad</u>

Description: A light dish of quinoa, cucumber, cherry tomatoes, olives, and feta cheese with a lemon-oregano vinaigrette.

Size of Serving: 2

Preparation Time: 15 minutes

Ingredients:

- 1 cup quinoa,

- chopped cucumber,
- diced Kalamata olives,
- rinsed cherry tomatoes,
- sliced Feta cheese,
- and crumbled lemon-oregano vinaigrette

Preparation Guide:

1. Quinoa, cucumber, cherry tomatoes, olives, and feta cheese should all be combined in a dish.
2. Add a lemon-oregano vinaigrette drizzle and toss to mix.

Hot Sweet Potato and Black Bean Bowl

Description: Quinoa, roasted sweet potatoes, cilantro, and lime drizzle combine to create a filling dish.

Size of Serving: 2

Preparation Time: 25 minutes

Ingredients:

- One cup of washed quinoa
- Cooked or canned black beans
- Sweet potatoes, chopped, cumin, and chili powder
- chopped fresh cilantro with lime juice

Preparation Guide:

1. Roast sweet potatoes until they become soft, adding cumin and chile powder.
2. Heat up some more chili powder with black beans in a saucepan.

3. Put quinoa, roasted sweet potatoes, and spicy black beans in bowls. Drizzle with lime-cilantro sauce.

Peanut Tofu Bowl with Thai Influence

Description: A dish of crunchy tofu, stir-fried veggies, brown rice, and a tasty peanut sauce with an Asian influence.

Size of Serving: 2

Preparation Time: 25 minutes

Ingredients:

- One cup cooked brown rice
- Crispy tofu that has been diced and sautéed
- Stir-fried mixed veggies (carrots, broccoli, and bell peppers) with seasonings of soy sauce, ginger, and garlic
- Peanut butter

Preparation Guide:

1. Follow the cooking directions on the package for brown rice.
2. Stir-fry mixed veggies with soy sauce, ginger, and garlic after the tofu has been sautéed until crispy.
3. Put stir-fried veggies, brown rice, and crispy tofu in bowls. Pour on some peanut sauce.

Quinoa Bowl with Lemon Garlic Shrimp

Description: A crisp and refreshing dish of quinoa, cherry tomatoes, arugula, and lemon-garlic shrimp, all tossed in a light vinaigrette.

Size of Serving: 2

Preparation Time: 15 minutes

Ingredients:

- 1 cup washed quinoa
- Deveined shrimp sautéed in garlic and lemon
- Half a cherry tomato
- Lettuce
- Vinaigrette with lemon

Preparation Guide:

1. Garlic and lemon should be sautéed until shrimp are done.
2. Quinoa, shrimp, cherry tomatoes, and arugula should all be combined in a dish.
3. Pour a lemon vinaigrette over it.

Chickpea and Couscous Moroccan Bowl

Description: A fragrant bowl of couscous, roasted veggies, spicy chickpeas, and a drizzle of mint yogurt.

Serving Size: Two

Preparation Time: 25 minutes

Ingredients:

- One cup of cooked couscous
- Moroccan-flavored canned or cooked chickpeas
- roasted veggies (zucchini, eggplant, and bell peppers)
- Greek yogurt, chopped fresh mint

Preparation Guide:

1. Cook the couscous as directed on the packet.
2. Chickpeas are sautéed till cooked with Moroccan spices.
3. Toss roasted veggies with couscous.
4. Top bowls with spicy chickpeas, couscous-vegetable mix, and mint-yogurt sauce.

Quinoa and Pesto Chicken Bowl

Description: A protein-rich dish with cherry tomatoes, quinoa, grilled chicken, and a sprinkle of basil pesto.

Preparation Time: 20 minutes

Ingredients:

- 1 cup washed quinoa
- Half a basil pesto, cut cherry tomatoes,
- and grilled chicken breast

Preparation Guide:

1. After the chicken is cooked through, slice it.
2. Place the quinoa, cherry tomatoes, and sliced chicken in a bowl.
3. Pour pesto basilico over it.

Brown Rice Bowl with Sesame Ginger Tofu

Description: Brown rice, stir-fried veggies, sesame ginger tofu, and a sesame-soy sauce combine in this Asian-inspired bowl.

Size of Serving: 2

Preparation Time: 25 minutes

Ingredients:

- One cup cooked brown rice
- Cubed and sautéed firm tofu with a sesame ginger marinade
- Stir-fried mixed veggies (carrots, bell peppers, and snow peas)
- Soy-sesame dressing

Preparation Guide:

1. Follow the cooking directions on the package for brown rice.
2. Use a sesame ginger marinade to sauté tofu until browned.
3. Mix veggies and stir-fry in soy sauce.
4. Put stir-fried veggies, brown rice, and sesame ginger tofu in bowls. Pour sesame-soy dressing over.

With their array of tastes, textures, and nutritional advantages, these one-pot superfood lunch bowls are tasty and easy choices for a filling and healthy noon meal. Savor the nutritious deliciousness and simplicity of preparation of these substantial lunch bowls!

Chapter 4

Dinners for Holistic Wellness

<u>Stir-fried Quinoa with Veggies</u>

Description: A satisfying and well-balanced supper with colorful veggies, quinoa, and a flavorful soy-ginger sauce combined in a nutrient-rich stir-fry.

Size of Serving: 4

Preparation Time: 20 minutes

Ingredients:

- One-cup quinoa
- mixed veggies, including carrots, broccoli, and bell peppers
- three tsp of soy sauce
- 1 tsp finely chopped ginger

Preparation Guide:

1. Stir-fry mixed veggies in a wok until they become tender.
2. Toss the cooked quinoa with the minced ginger and soy sauce in the pan.

<u>Lemon-Dill Sauced Baked Salmon</u>

Description: A heart-healthy supper of roasted sweet potatoes and steamed asparagus accompanied by baked salmon fillets in a zesty lemon-dill sauce.

Serving Size: Two; 10-minute prep

Ingredients:

- 2 fillets of salmon
- Juiced one lime
- freshly sliced dill
- Diced sweet potatoes
- spears of asparagus

Preparation Guide:

1. Bake the salmon with chopped dill and lemon juice after preheating the oven.
2. Steam asparagus until it's soft, then roast sweet potatoes into dice.

Curry with Lentils and Vegetables

Description: A hearty and fragrant curry made with lentils and vegetables that is served over brown rice and is a great way to receive important nutrients and plant-based protein.

Size of Serving: 4

Cooking Period: Half an hour

Ingredients:

- cup of lentils
- A mixture of bell peppers, zucchini, and carrots
- One coconut milk can
- Curry seasonings (coriander, cumin, and turmeric)

Preparation Guide:

1. As directed on the box, prepare the lentils.
2. Stir-fry a mixture of veggies in a saucepan with coconut milk and curry powder.

3. After the veggies are soft, simmer them and serve them over prepared brown rice.

Salad with Mediterranean Chickpeas

Description: A salad with cucumber, feta cheese, cherry tomatoes, and chickpeas dressed with a lemon-olive oil vinaigrette that is light and delicious.

Serving Size: Two

15 minutes for preparation

Ingredients:

- 1 can rinsed and drained chickpeas
- Diced Feta cheese, chopped cucumber, cherry tomatoes, and crumbled
- Olive oil and lemon dressing

Preparation Guide:

1. Chickpeas, cucumber, cherry tomatoes, and feta cheese should all be combined in a dish.
2. Add a little drizzle of lemon-olive oil dressing and gently mix.

Stir-fried Teriyaki Tofu with Veggies

Description: Served over brown rice, this dish is a tasty and high-protein stir-fry cooked with tofu, broccoli, and bell peppers in a homemade teriyaki sauce.

Size of Serving: 4

Preparation Time: 20 minutes

Ingredients:

- One block of diced and pressed tofu
- Frolicking broccoli
- Diced bell peppers
- cooked brown rice
- Tiramisu cooked from scratch

Preparation Guide:

1. Cubed tofu is sautéed till golden brown.
2. Stir in the homemade teriyaki sauce after adding the bell peppers and broccoli.
3. Place on top of warm brown rice.

Black beans and Quinoa Stuffed Bell Peppers

Description: Perfectly cooked bell peppers packed with quinoa, black beans, corn, and spices, garnished with avocado and cilantro.

Size of Serving: 3

Cooking Period: Half an hour

Ingredients:

- 1 cup cooked quinoa, 3 bell peppers, drained and washed corn kernels, and drained black beans.
- Toppings: avocado and cilantro

Preparation Guide:

1. Bell peppers should be baked after preheating the oven.
2. Combine cooked quinoa, corn, and black beans.

3. Once the bell peppers are soft, stuff them with the quinoa mixture and bake them.

4. Add sliced avocado and cilantro on top.

Pasta with Lemon Garlic Shrimp

Description: Serves well over whole-grain spaghetti, this meal is a light and tasty pasta with shrimp, cherry tomatoes, and spinach in a lemon-garlic sauce.

Size of Serving: 2

Preparation Time: 15 minutes

Ingredients:

- One-half pound of peeled and deveined shrimp
- Grain-free spaghetti
- Half a cherry tomato
- new spinach
- Garlic and lemon sauce

Preparation Guide:

1. Follow the directions on the package to cook the whole-grain spaghetti.
2. Sauté shrimp in a lemon-garlic sauce with cherry tomatoes and spinach.
3. Over cooked pasta, serve shrimp mixture.

Enchiladas with Sweet Potatoes and Black Beans

Description: Baked enchiladas stuffed with a flavorful blend of sweet potatoes, black beans, and spices, covered with melted cheese and enchilada sauce.

Size of Serving: 4

Preparation Time: 25 minutes

Ingredients:

- Two sweet potatoes, baked and chopped
- One can of mashed black beans
- Grains-based tortillas
- Mexican sauce
- Cheese shreds for the garnish

Preparation Guide:

1. Sweet potatoes should be roasted until soft.
2. Mash black beans with roasted sweet potatoes.
3. After stuffing tortillas with the black bean and sweet potato mixture, roll them up, and put them on a baking tray.
4. Add shredded cheese and enchilada sauce on top, and bake until bubbling.

Grilled Chicken Salad with Mediterranean Flavors

Description: A salad with grilled chicken, cherry tomatoes, olives, feta cheese, and a balsamic vinaigrette that's light and full of protein.

Size of Serving: 2

Preparation Time: 15 minutes

Ingredients:

- sliced and grilled chicken breasts
- mixed greens for salad
- sliced Feta cheese, chopped Kalamata olives, cherry tomatoes, and crumbled balsamic vinaigrette

Preparation Guide:

1. After the chicken breasts are cooked through, slice them.
2. Salad greens, cherry tomatoes, olives, and sliced chicken should all be combined in a dish.
3. Top with crumbled feta cheese and a balsamic vinaigrette drizzle.

<u>Primavera Spaghetti Squash</u>

Description: A low-carb substitute for classic pasta, marinara sauce-tossed spaghetti squash is topped with grated Parmesan and sautéed veggies.

Size of Serving: 3

Preparation Time: 45 minutes

Ingredients:

- 1 halved and seeded spaghetti squash
- mixed veggies, including cherry tomatoes, bell peppers, and zucchini
- Toscana sauce

- grated parmigiano as a garnish

Preparation Guide:

1. Roast the halves of the spaghetti squash until soft.
2. Mix veggies in a skillet and stir with marinara sauce.
3. After cooking the spaghetti squash, scrape it with a fork to make "noodles" and add the veggie mixture on top.
4. Before serving, top with grated Parmesan cheese.

These supper dishes combine a range of tastes, textures, and nutrient-dense foods to produce filling and nutritious meals that provide a holistic approach to wellbeing. Savor the balance and nutrition that these recipes will offer to your dinner table!

Flavorful Superfood Stir-Fries

Rainbow Stir-Fry with Quinoa and Vegetables

Description: A savory soy-ginger sauce is combined with colorful quinoa, bell peppers, broccoli, and carrots to create a vibrant, filling dish that is high in nutrients.

Size of Serving: 2

Preparation Time: 15 minutes

Ingredients:

- 1 cup of quinoa, cooked
- Sliced bell peppers in a mixture
- Frolicking broccoli
- For the sauce, combine carrots, julienned Soy sauce, ginger, and garlic.

Preparation Guide:

1. Stir-fry the carrots, broccoli, and bell peppers in a wok until they are crisp-tender.
2. To the pan, add the cooked quinoa.
3. Combine the garlic, ginger, and soy sauce in a bowl. Pour over the veggies and quinoa, tossing to cover well.

Stir-fried Teriyaki Tofu with Bok Choy

Description: A tasty stir-fry with colorful bok choy and crunchy tofu, topped with a housemade teriyaki sauce and served over brown rice for a filling and hearty meal.

Size of Serving: 2

Preparation Time: 15 minutes

Ingredients:

- Cooked Teriyaki sauce (soy sauce, honey, garlic, and ginger),
- chopped brown rice,
- diced and pan-fried bok choy, and firm tofu

Preparation Guide:

1. Fry tofu in a pan until crispy.
2. Stir-fry the bok choy in the same pan until it wilts.
3. After adding the cooked brown rice, cover the mixture with teriyaki sauce and toss to thoroughly incorporate.

Power Stir-Fry with Kale and Chickpeas

Description: A colorful and high-protein dish made with kale, chickpeas, cherry tomatoes, and quinoa combined in a lemon-tahini sauce, this stir-fry is packed with nutrients.

Serving Size: Two

Preparation Time: 15 minutes

Ingredients:

- half a quinoa, cooked cherry tomatoes,
- diced and destemmed chickpeas,
- and prepared lemon-tahini vinaigrette

Preparation Guide:

1. Eat the kale raw until it wilts.
2. To the pan, add the cherry tomatoes and chickpeas.
3. Add the cooked quinoa and toss to thoroughly combine, then sprinkle with the lemon-tahini dressing.

Hot Stir-fried Shrimp with Asparagus

Description: Succulent shrimp, crisp asparagus, and bell peppers are stir-fried in a spicy garlic and soy sauce and served over rice noodles in this flavorful dish.

Size of Serving: 2

20 minutes for preparation

Ten minutes for cooking

Ingredients.

- Peeled and deveined shrimp
- Trimmed and sliced asparagus;
- thinly sliced bell peppers; cooked rice noodles
- hot soy-garlic sauce

Preparation Guide:

1. Shrimp should be sautéed until pink and opaque.
2. Add bell peppers and asparagus to the pan.
3. Add the cooked rice noodles and stir with a hot sauce made of garlic and soy.

Broccoli and Sesame Ginger Chicken Stir-Fry

Description: Served over steaming jasmine rice, this classic stir-fry has succulent chicken, broccoli florets, and snap peas, all covered in a delicious sesame-ginger sauce.

Size of Serving: 2

Preparation Time: 15 minutes

Ingredients:

- Thickly cut chicken breast
- Frolicking broccoli
- Quick peas
- Rice with jasmine steamed
- Ginger-sesame sauce

Preparation Guide:

1. Cook the chicken thoroughly by sautéing it.
2. Add snap peas and broccoli to the pan.

3. Over the mixture, drizzle the sesame-ginger sauce and toss until thoroughly covered.
4. Accompany with steaming jasmine rice.

Stir-fried Veggies with Turmeric and Coconut

Description: A healthy and anti-inflammatory stir-fry made with quinoa, tofu, and a rainbow of colorful veggies that is flavored with coconut and turmeric.

Size of Serving: 2

Preparation Time: 15 minutes

Ingredients:

- Pan-fried, cubed tofu
- Vegetable mixture (peas, carrots, and bell peppers)
- Cooked quinoa
- Curry powder and coconut milk

Preparation Guide:

1. Sauté mixed veggies until they are crisp-tender.
2. Toss in the cooked quinoa and pan-fried tofu.
3. After adding a drizzle of coconut sauce and turmeric, mix to coat evenly.

Stir-fried Chicken with Cashews and Pineapples

Description: A delightful blend of sweet and savory flavors, this stir-fry is served over brown rice and includes juicy pineapple chunks, bell peppers, cashews, and delicate chicken all coated in a delicious soy-ginger sauce.

Size of Serving: 2

Preparation Time: 15 minutes

Ingredients:

- pieces of pineapple,
- thinly sliced chicken breast
- Sweet peppers and chopped cashews
- Ginger-soy glaze

Preparation Guide:

1. Cook the chicken thoroughly by sautéing it.
2. To the pan, add the pineapple, bell peppers, and cashews.
3. Over the mixture, drizzle the soy-ginger glaze and swirl until well covered.
4. Put on top of brown rice.

Stir-fried Curry with Cauliflower and Chickpeas

Description: A filling and fragrant meal of tasty stir-fried cauliflower florets, chickpeas, and spinach cooked in a coconut curry sauce, served over basmati rice.

Size of Serving: 2

Preparation Time: 20 minutes

Ingredients:

- Fresh cauliflower
- Curry beans, cooked Sprouts
- Cubed basmati rice
- Curry sauce with coconut.

Preparation Guide:

1. Cauliflower should be cooked until gently browned.
2. Stir in the chickpeas and spinach.
3. After adding the coconut curry sauce, boil the veggies until they are soft. Put on top of basmati rice.

Spicy Garlic and Lemon Shrimp Stir-Fry

Description: For a low-carb option, try this zesty and light stir-fry with shrimp, snow peas, and bell peppers mixed in a lemon-garlic sauce and served over cauliflower rice.

Size of Serving: 2

20 minutes for preparation

Ten minutes for cooking

Ingredients.

- Peeled and deveined shrimp
- White peas
- Cooked bell peppers, sliced cauliflower rice
- Garlic and lemon sauce

Preparation Guide:

1. Shrimp should be sautéed until pink and opaque.
2. Toss in the snow peas and bell peppers.

3. Over the mixture, drizzle the lemon-garlic sauce and toss until thoroughly covered.
4. Put on top of cauliflower rice.

Stir-fried Vegetables with Ginger Soy Tofu

Description: A hearty and filling stir-fry made with tofu, broccoli, and bell peppers that is vegetarian and laced with a ginger-soy marinade. It is served over brown rice.

Size of Serving: 2

Preparation Time: 15 minutes

Ingredients:

- Cubed and pan-fried firm tofu
- Frolicking broccoli
- Sliced bell peppers thinly
- cooked brown rice
- Soy-ginger marinade

Preparation Guide:

1. Fried tofu in a pan till brown and crispy.
2. Broccoli and bell peppers should be sautéed until crisp-tender.
3. Combine veggies and pan-fried tofu with a ginger-soy marinade. Put on top of brown rice.

These savory stir-fry recipes for superfoods provide a range of colorful and nourishing choices, combining a variety of ingredients and tastes to make filling meals. Every stir-fry has a different touch, from protein-rich tofu to tender shrimp, making eating healthfully a delightful experience. Savor the healthful benefits of these stir-fried superfoods!

Wholesome Grain and Protein Combos

Black Bean and Quinoa Power Bowl

Description: A healthy and high-protein dish made with quinoa, black beans, avocado, and a zesty lime dressing, this bowl is full of nutrients.

Size of Serving: 2

Preparation Time: 15 minutes

Ingredients:

- One cup of cooked quinoa
- One can of well cleaned and emptied black beans
- 1 sliced avocado
- fresh cilantro, chopped; lime dressing (lime juice, olive oil, salt)

Preparation Guide:

1. Put the cooked quinoa, black beans, and avocado slices in a bowl.
2. Add a lime dressing drizzle and some fresh cilantro as a garnish.

Quinoa Bowl with Chickpeas and Spinach

A filling combination of grains and proteins, this dish has quinoa, chickpeas, sautéed spinach, and a tahini dressing.

Size of Serving: 2

Preparation Time: 20 minutes

Ingredients:

- One cup of cooked quinoa
- One can of washed and drained chickpeas

Preparation Guide:

1. Add fresh spinach and sautéed it with a tahini dressing (tahini, lemon juice, garlic, and salt).
2. In a bowl, mix the cooked quinoa, sautéed spinach, and chickpeas.
3. Pour over tahini dressing and mix until well covered.

Stuffed Bell Peppers with Lentil and Brown Rice

Description: A filling and high-protein dish made with wholesome bell peppers filled with a blend of brown rice, lentils, tomatoes, and spices.

Serving Size: 4 pieces

20 minutes for preparation

40 minutes for cooking

Ingredients:

- 1 cup cooked brown rice
- One cup cooked lentils with halved and deseed Bell peppers

- chopped tomato
- Finely chopped onion; minced garlic
- Spices (pepper, salt, paprika, and cumin)

Preparation Guide:

1. Turn the oven on to 375°F, or 190°C.
2. Cooked brown rice, lentils, diced tomatoes, chopped onion, minced garlic, and spices should all be combined in a bowl.
3. Bake the filled bell pepper halves for 30 to 40 minutes, or until the peppers are soft.

Quinoa and Salmon Salad

Description: A light salad with quinoa, mixed greens, and a lemon vinaigrette that has grilled salmon and provides a good balance of grains and protein.

Size of Serving: 2

Ten minutes for cooking

Ingredients:

- 2 fillets of salmon
- One cup of cooked quinoa
- Various greens
- Half a cherry tomato
- Honey, Dijon mustard, olive oil, and lemon juice make up a lemon vinaigrette.

Preparation Guide:

1. Salmon fillets should be cooked thoroughly on a grill.

2. Put the cooked quinoa, cherry tomatoes, and mixed greens in a bowl.
3. Add grilled salmon on top and dress with a lemon vinaigrette.

Quinoa Bowl with Sweet Potatoes and Turkey

Description: A filling and healthy dish consisting of quinoa, roasted sweet potatoes, ground turkey, and a flavorful herb dressing served in a substantial bowl.

Serving Size: Two

20-minute prep

Cooking Period: Half an hour

Ingredients:

- One cup of cooked quinoa
- 1 pound of turkey meat
- Sweet potatoes cut into cubes and peels
- fresh herbs (thyme, rosemary)
- Olive oil.
- To taste, add salt and pepper.

Preparation Guide:

1. Sweet potatoes should be roasted till soft with olive oil, salt, pepper, and fresh herbs.
2. Cook the ground turkey in a pan until browned.
3. Ground turkey, roasted sweet potatoes, and cooked quinoa should all be combined in a dish.

Brown Rice Stir-Fry with Tofu and Veggies

Description: A tasty plant-based protein and grain combination made with tofu, various veggies, and brown rice stir-fried in a delicious soy-ginger sauce.

Size of Serving: 2

Prepare Duration: 15 minutes.

Preparation Time: 15 minutes

Ingredients:

- 1 cup cooked brown rice
- Tight tofu, mashed
- Broccoli, bell peppers, carrots, and mixed veggies with sliced Soy-ginger sauce (soy sauce, ginger, garlic, and sesame oil)

Preparation Guide:

1. Fry the tofu in a pan or skillet until it becomes brown.
2. Stir-fry the cut veggies until they become soft.
3. Add the cooked brown rice and soy-ginger sauce, stirring to thoroughly blend.

Chicken Bowl with Quinoa and Pesto

Description: A tasty and protein-rich dish of quinoa, grilled chicken marinated in pesto, cherry tomatoes, and basil pesto dressing.

Size of Serving: 2

Preparation Time: 15 minutes

Ingredients:

- 1 cup cooked quinoa; marinated chicken breast in pesto;
- Half a jar of basil pesto dressing and cherry tomatoes

Preparation Guide:

1. Grill the pesto-marinated chicken breast until it's done.
2. Place the cooked quinoa, cherry tomatoes, and grilled chicken slices into a bowl.
3. After adding a drizzle of basil pesto dressing, toss to coat well.

Wild Rice Pilaf with Shrimp

Description: A delicious and high-protein pilaf made with wild rice, tender shrimp, peas, and a sauce of lemon garlic butter.

Size of Serving: 2

Cooking Period: Half an hour

Ingredients:

- 1 cup cooked wild rice; peeled and deveined shrimp
- Green beans
- Sauce made with butter, garlic, and lemon juice and lemon juice.

Preparation Guide:

1. Sauté shrimp in a pan until they are cooked through and pink.
2. To the skillet, add the cooked wild rice and peas.

3. Pour in the lemon-garlic butter sauce and stir to mix thoroughly.

Breakfast Bowl with Egg and Quinoa.

Description: For a healthy start to the day, try this protein-rich breakfast bowl that has sautéed spinach, quinoa, scrambled eggs, and feta cheese.

Size of Serving: 2

Preparation Time: 15 minutes

Ingredients:

- 1 cup cooked quinoa, scrambled eggs,
- shredded Feta cheese, sautéed spinach, and fresh

Preparation Guide:

1. Put cooked quinoa, scrambled eggs, and sautéed spinach in a bowl.
2. Add some crumbled feta cheese on top.

Stew with Barley and Beef

Description: A filling and high-protein one-pot dish made with lean beef, barley, veggies, and fragrant spices, this stew is robust and satisfying.

Size of Serving: 4

20 minutes for preparation

Cooking Period: 60 Minutes

Ingredients:

- Cubbed lean beef stew meat
- Barley pearl
- Celery, onions, carrots, and diced
- Beef consommé
- Add the bay leaves, garlic, minced thyme, salt, and pepper.

Preparation Guide:

1. Brown the cubes of beef with chopped garlic in a big saucepan.
2. Stir in the barley, beef broth, seasonings, and chopped veggies.
3. Simmer for one hour, or until the flavors combine and the meat becomes soft.

These nutritious grain and protein combinations provide a range of tastes, textures, and health advantages. These dishes offer well-balanced and fulfilling meals that support a nutritious and healthful diet, regardless of your preference for lean meats or plant-based foods. Savor the healthful benefits of these delectable combos!

Oven-Baked Superfood Delights

Kale and Sweet Potato Salad

Description: A nutrient-dense dish of crispy kale and roasted sweet potatoes combined with feta cheese, quinoa, and a tangy lemon vinaigrette.

Size of Serving: 2
Preparation Time: 25 minutes
Ingredients:

- One sweet potato, diced and peeled
- Two cups of chopped and removed stemmed kale
- 1 cup of quinoa, cooked
- Half a cup of crumbled feta cheese
- Lemon vinaigrette (salt, pepper, Dijon mustard, lemon juice, and olive oil)

Preparation Guide:

1. Sweet potatoes should be tossed with salt, pepper, and olive oil. Preheat oven to 400°F (200°C) and roast 20 minutes.
2. Toss the kale with the sweet potatoes on the baking sheet, then roast for a further five minutes.
3. Add the feta, quinoa, and roasted veggies to a dish. Pour a lemon vinaigrette over it.

Quinoa Pilaf-Studded Baked Salmon

Description: Baked salmon fillets with spinach, tomatoes, and a lemon-herb drizzle are served on quinoa pilaf in this tasty and omega-3-rich recipe.

Size of Serving: 2
Preparation Time: 20 minutes
Ingredients:

- 2 fillets of salmon
- One cup of cooked quinoa

- Scoop of spinach
- Half a cherry tomato
- Lemon-herb drizzle (garlic, thyme, olive oil, lemon juice, salt, and pepper)

Preparation Guide:

1. Salt, pepper, and olive oil are used to season fish. Bake 15 to 18 minutes at 375°F (190°C).
2. Cook the spinach and cherry tomatoes in a pan. Add cooked quinoa and stir.
3. Drizzle fish with lemon-herb sauce and serve it over quinoa pilaf.

Brussels Sprouts Glazed with Turmeric

Description: A tasty and anti-inflammatory side dish made of oven-baked Brussels sprouts covered in a golden turmeric glaze.

Size of Serving: 4
Preparation Time: 25 minutes
Ingredients:

- One pound of halved Brussels sprouts
- Two tsp of olive oil
- One tsp of turmeric
- Add pepper and salt to taste.

Preparation Guide:

1. Add salt, pepper, turmeric, and olive oil to Brussels sprouts and toss.

2. Roast for 20 to 25 minutes at 400°F (200°C), or until brown and crispy.

Stuffed Bell Peppers with Quinoa

Description: Vibrant bell peppers filled with quinoa, black beans, corn, and spices—a superfood blend—that are cooked to perfection and garnished with avocado salsa.

Size of Serving: 4
20 minutes for preparation
Cooking Period: Half an hour
Ingredients:

- 4 cleaned, halved bell peppers
- One can of rinsed and drained black beans and one cup of cooked quinoa
- One cup of kernel corn
- Seasoning for tacos, to taste
- Avocado with tomatoes, red onion, cilantro, and lime juice is a salsa.

Preparation Guide:

1. Combine the taco seasoning, cooked quinoa, black beans, and corn.
2. After stuffing bell peppers with the quinoa mixture, bake for 25 to 30 minutes at 375°F (190°C).
3. Before serving, spread avocado salsa on top.

Baked Chicken with Lemon Herbs

Description: Baked to perfection, succulent chicken breasts marinated in a zesty lemon herb combination served with roasted veggies on the side.

Size of Serving: 2
Preparation Time: 25 minutes
Ingredients:

- Two hens' breasts
- Two tsp of olive oil
- Zest and juice of lemons
- The fresh herbs (oregano, thyme, and rosemary)
- Add pepper and salt to taste.
- a variety of veggies for roasting, including bell peppers, broccoli, and carrots

Preparation Guide:

1. For at least fifteen minutes, marinate chicken breasts in a mixture of olive oil, lemon zest,
2. lemon juice, fresh herbs, salt, and pepper.
3. Bake chicken for 20 to 25 minutes at 400°F (200°C).
4. Roast the veggies until they are soft with the chicken.

Baked Eggplant with a Mediterranean Flavor

Description: A delicious and filling dish made of sliced eggplant roasted to perfection with tomatoes, feta cheese, and Mediterranean seasonings.

Size of Serving: 4

Preparation Time: 35 minutes
Ingredients:

- 1/2 cup feta cheese,
- 2 cups tomatoes,
- 1 big eggplant, chopped garlic powder, oregano, salt, and pepper.

Preparation Guide:

1. Place the slices of eggplant in a baking dish. Season with garlic powder, oregano, salt, and pepper.
2. Drizzle with olive oil.
3. Add sliced tomatoes and crumbled feta on top. Bake for 30 to 35 minutes at 375°F (190°C).

Quinoa Salad with Pesto Infusion

Description: A colorful side dish of quinoa salad flavored with homemade pesto, cherry tomatoes, mozzarella, and pine nuts that is cooked to perfection.

Size of Serving: 4
Prep Time: 20 minutes
Ingredients:

- Half a mozzarella ball,
- cooked cherry tomatoes,
- and one cup of quinoa
- Olive oil, basil, garlic, pine nuts, Parmesan,
- and homemade pesto

Preparation Guide:

1. Combine cooked quinoa with homemade pesto, mozzarella balls, and cherry tomatoes.
2. Place in a baking dish and bake for 15 to 20 minutes at 375°F (190°C).

<u>Stuffed Mushrooms with Superfood</u>

Description: Baked to perfection, mushroom caps filled with a superfood blend of quinoa, spinach, and feta cheese make a flavorful and nutrient-dense appetizer.

Size of Serving: 4
Preparation Time: 25 minutes
Ingredients:

- 16 big mushroom caps,
- 1 cup boiled spinach,
- 1 cup cleaned quinoa,
- 1/2 cup minced feta cheese, and crumbled
- Garlic, salt, pepper, and olive oil

Preparation Guide:

1. Add chopped spinach to olive oil-sautéd garlic and simmer until wilted.
2. Combine the cooked quinoa, crumbled feta, and sautéed spinach in a bowl.

3. Place the quinoa mixture inside the mushroom caps and bake for 20 to 25 minutes at 375°F (190°C).

Crunchy Kale Chips

Description: Crispy and savory superfood chips made from oven-baked kale leaves seasoned with nutritional yeast, olive oil, and a touch of cayenne.

Size of Serving: 2
Preparation Time: 15 minutes
Ingredients:

- 1 bunch of kale with ripped leaves and stems
- Two tsp of olive oil
- Cayenne, nutritional yeast, salt, and pepper

Preparation Guide:

1. Combine olive oil, nutritional yeast, cayenne, salt, and pepper with the kale leaves.
2. Place on a baking sheet and bake for 10 to 15 minutes, or until crispy, at 350°F/175°C.

Baked Tofu with Coconut Crumbs

Description: Crispy coconut crusted tofu cubes are cooked till golden and served with tangy and sweet mango salsa for a tropical twist.

Size of Serving: 4
Preparation Time: 25 minutes
Ingredients:

- One block of pressed and diced extra-firm tofu
- One cup of coconut shreds
- half a cup of crumbs
- Mango salsa made with lime juice, cilantro, red onion, and mango

Preparation Guide:

1. Mix the breadcrumbs with the shredded coconut.
   Tofu cubes should be coated in the coconut mixture and baked for 20 to 25 minutes at 375°F (190°C).
2. Mango salsa should be served alongside.

These deliciously nutritious oven-baked superfoods come in a variety of flavors. Every recipe offers a tasty and healthful way to include nutrient-dense foods in your meals, from protein-rich quinoa dishes to roasted veggies. Savor this delicious and nutritious culinary experience with these oven-baked delights!

Chapter 5

Snacks and Treats for Guilt-Free Indulgence

<u>Date Energy Bites with Almonds</u>

Description: Bite-sized energy balls filled with a combination of dates, almonds, and a touch of cinnamon, wrapped in a guilt-free delight.

Size of Serving: 10 Bits

15 minutes for preparation

Ingredients:

- cup of almonds
- one cup of pitted dates
- half a teaspoon of cinnamon

Preparation Guide:

1. In a food processor, pulse almonds, dates, and cinnamon until a sticky paste forms.
2. After forming the mixture into bite-sized balls, chill it for a minimum of half an hour.

<u>Berry Parfait with Greek Yogurt</u>

Description: A delicious and high-protein parfait that combines Greek yogurt, fresh berries, and granola.

Serving Size: One;

5-Minute Preparation

Ingredients:

- Greek yogurt, one cup
- Strawberries, blueberries, and raspberries are mixed berries.
- Oatmeal

Preparation Guide:

1. Arrange Greek yogurt, granola, and fresh berries in a glass.
2. Continue layering, then savor this guilt-free parfait.

Roasted Chickpeas with Spices

Description: Roasted chickpeas combined with a variety of spices make for a crispy, flavorful, guilt-free snack that replaces typical nibbles.

Portion Size: Two Cups

Ten minutes to prepare.

40 minutes for cooking

Ingredients:

- Two cans of rinsed and drained chickpeas
- Two tsp of olive oil
- One tsp cumin
- One tsp of paprika
- Half a teaspoon of chili powder

Preparation Guide:

1. Toss chickpeas with spices and olive oil.
2. Bake at 400°F (200°C) for forty minutes, turning once throughout that time.

Strawberries Dipped in Dark Chocolate

Description: A delightful and antioxidant-rich dessert made with juicy strawberries covered in dark chocolate, all without the guilt.

Size of Serving: ten strawberries

15 minutes for preparation

Five minutes for cooking

Ingredients:

- ten cleaned and dehydrated strawberries
- 50 milligrams of dark chocolate chips

Preparation Guide:

1. Put dark chocolate in a dish that is safe to microwave.
2. After dipping each strawberry into the molten chocolate, set them aside to cool on a dish lined with paper.

Hummus-Stuffed Veggie Sticks

Description: A filling and nutritious snack that comes with homemade hummus and vibrant veggie sticks.

Size of Serving: 2

Ten minutes to prepare.

Ingredients:

- Bell pepper, cucumber,
- and carrot sticks Hummus.

Preparation Guide:

1. Chop veggies into sticks.
2. Enjoy this crispy, guilt-free snack by dipping the vegetable sticks into hummus.

Almond Butter and Apple Nachos

Description: Apple slices with almond butter poured over them, topped with granola and a dash of cinnamon, make up this sweet and crispy treat.

Serving Size: 1

10-minute prep

Ingredients:

- One finely cut apple
- Double-stick of almond butter
- Granola Cinnamon to Add to Food

Preparation Guide:

1. Place sliced apples on a platter.
2. Sprinkle with granola, drizzle with almond butter, and dust with cinnamon.

Tomato and Avocado Salsa

Description: Served with whole-grain tortilla chips, this crisp and nutrient-dense salsa has diced avocado and tomatoes.

Portion Size: Two Cups

Ten minutes to prepare.

Ingredients:

- 2 sliced avocados
- Half a cup of cherry tomatoes
- sliced red onion, finely
- chopped fresh cilantro
- Lime juice, to taste with salt and pepper

Preparation Guide:

- In a bowl, mix together chopped avocado, tomatoes, red onion, and cilantro.
- Add pepper, salt, and lime juice for seasoning. Accompany with whole-grain taco chips.

Hummus and Cucumber Bites

Description: A simple and cool snack consisting of cucumber slices with cherry tomatoes and hummus on top.

Size of Serving: 2

Ten minutes to prepare.

Ingredients:

- 1 sliced cucumber with hummus
- Half a cherry tomato

Preparation Guide:

1. Arrange slices of cucumber on a platter.

2. Place a halved cherry tomato and some hummus on top of each slice.

Almond Trail Mix

Description: A customized blend of nuts, seeds, and dried fruits that makes for a crunchy, gratifying, guilt-free trail mix.

Cup of serving size

Five minutes to prepare

Ingredients:

- dark chocolate chips,
- pumpkin seeds,
- walnuts,
- almonds,
- and dried cranberries

Preparation Guide:

- In a bowl, combine all divide into portions the size of snacks for an easy and wholesome treat.

Bits of Frozen Bananas

Description: A guilt-free dessert consisting of frozen banana slices coated in yogurt and wrapped in crushed almonds.

One serving size

15 minutes for preparation

Ingredients:

- Greek yogurt, sliced banana
- Crushed nuts (pistachios, almonds) Preparation Guide:
- Dredge slices of banana in Greek yogurt.
- Before serving, roll in chopped nuts and put in the freezer for at least two hours.

In addition to satisfying your desires, these guilt-free snacks and sweets come in a range of tastes and textures and are healthy, nourishing substitutes for conventional pleasures. Savor these mouthwatering choices without sacrificing flavor or health!

Superfood Energy Bites

<u>Energy Bites with Almond Joy</u>

Description: Delectable and stimulating snack, these energy bites are made with almonds, coconut, and dark chocolate.

Meal Size: Twelve Bits

15 minutes for preparation

Ingredients:

- cup of almonds
- 1/2 cup of coconut shreds
- 1/4 cup chips made with dark chocolate
- Double-stick of almond butter
- One spoonful of honey

Preparation Guide:

1. Process almonds in a food processor until they are coarsely chopped.

2. Add the almond butter, honey, dark chocolate chips, and shredded coconut. Once the mixture is thoroughly mixed, pulse.
3. Before serving, roll the mixture into bite-sized balls and place in the refrigerator for at least 30 minutes.

Energy Bites with Matcha Bliss

Description: A quick description of these bite-sized, delicious balls of matcha, almonds, and dates is that they provide a burst of energy.

Size of Serving: 10 Bits

20 minutes for preparation

Ingredients:

- cup of almonds
- half a cup of pitted dates
- One tablespoon powdered matcha
- One tsp of coconut oil
- 1/4 cup of coconut shreds (for rolling)

Preparation Guide:

1. Process almonds in a food processor until they are finely crushed.
2. Add coconut oil, matcha powder, and dates. Pulse to produce a sticky dough.
3. Form the mixture into small, bite-sized balls and roll them in coconut shreds.
4. Let it cool for a minimum of half an hour before serving.

Energy Bites with Cocoa Crunch

Description: A delicious energy bite with a crunch from the quinoa and chocolate combined with the dried fruits.

Serving Quantity: 15 pieces

15 minutes for preparation

Ingredients:

- Half a cup of cooked and cooled quinoa
- 1/4 cup of chopped almonds
- 1/4 cup of cranberries, dried
- Twice as much cocoa powder
- Double-stick of almond butter
- One spoonful of honey

Preparation Guide:

1. Cooked quinoa, sliced almonds, dried cranberries, cocoa powder, almond butter, and honey should all be combined in a dish.
2. After thoroughly mixing, form the mixture into little balls that may be eaten.
3. Let it cool for a minimum of half an hour before serving.

Protein Bites with Peanut Butter

Description: Rich tastes of peanut butter, oats, and chia seeds combine to create protein-rich energy pieces that make a filling and healthy snack.

Meal Size: Twelve Bits

15 minutes for preparation

Ingredients:

- Oats, rolled, one cup
- half a cup of peanut butter
- 1/4 cup of honey.
- 1/4 cup of protein powder (chocolate or vanilla)
- Two tsp of chia seeds

Preparation Guide:

1. Rolling oats, peanut butter, honey, protein powder, and chia seeds should all be combined in a dish.
2. Roll the dense dough into bite-sized balls after mixing.
3. Let it cool for a minimum of half an hour before serving.

<u>Almond Joy Bites with Turmeric</u>

Description: A blend of superfoods including coconut, almonds, and turmeric that creates a distinct anti-inflammatory energy bite.

Size of Serving: 10 Bits

20 minutes for preparation

Ingredients:

- cup of almonds
- 1/4 cup of coconut, shredded
- 1 tsp powdered turmeric
- Double-stick of almond butter
- One spoonful of honey

Preparation Guide:

1. Process almonds in a food processor until they are finely crushed.
2. Stir in the honey, almond butter, shredded coconut, and turmeric powder. Once the mixture is thoroughly mixed, pulse.
3. Before serving, roll the mixture into bite-sized balls and place in the refrigerator for at least 30 minutes.

Goji Berry and Chia Seed Bites

Description: Powerful energy bites loaded with superfoods like goji berries, almonds, and chia seeds that provide a high-nutrient, high-antioxidant snack.

Serving Quantity: 15 pieces

15 minutes for preparation

Ingredients:

1. Half a cup of chia seeds
2. Goji berries, 1/4 cup
3. cup of almonds
4. Double-stick of almond butter
5. 1/4 cup of honey.

Preparation Guide:

1. Chia seeds, goji berries, almonds, almond butter, and honey should all be combined in a dish.
2. After thoroughly mixing, form the mixture into little balls that may be eaten.
3. Let it cool for a minimum of half an hour before serving.

Almond-Blueberry Energy Bites

Description: Packed full of the health benefits of oats, almonds, and blueberries, these energy bites have a delicious crunch and sweetness ratio.

Meal Size: Twelve Bits

15 minutes for preparation

Ingredients:

- Half a cup of blueberries, dry
- cup of almonds
- Oats, half a cup rolled
- Double-stick of almond butter
- 1/4 cup of honey.

Preparation Guide:

1. Process the almonds, rolled oats, honey, almond butter, and dried blueberries in a food processor until well combined.
2. Before serving, roll the mixture into bite-sized balls and place in the refrigerator for at least 30 minutes.

Energy Bites with Spirulina and Dates

Description: A nutrient-dense, naturally sweetened energy bite with dates, almonds, and the superfood spirulina for a satisfying treat.

Size of Serving: 10 Bits

20 minutes for preparation

Ingredients:

- one cup of pitted dates
- one-half cup almonds
- One spoonful of powdered spirulina
- One tsp almond butter
- 1/4 cup of coconut shreds (for rolling)

Preparation Guide:

1. Process dates, almonds, spirulina powder, and almond butter in a food processor until a sticky dough develops.
2. Form the mixture into small, bite-sized balls and roll them in coconut shreds. Let it cool for a minimum of half an hour before serving.

Energy Bites with Pumpkin Pie Spice

Description: A tasty and festive energy bite with dates, pecans, and pumpkin pie spice that gives every mouthful a hint of the season.

Meal Size: Twelve Bits

15 minutes for preparation

Ingredients:

- Cup of pecans
- half a cup of pitted dates
- One teaspoon spice (pumpkin pie)
- One tsp almond butter
- Oats, 1/4 cup rolled

1. Process dates, almond butter, pumpkin pie spice, pecans, and rolled oats in a food processor until a sticky dough forms.
2. Before serving, roll the mixture into bite-sized balls and place in the refrigerator for at least 30 minutes.

Chocolate Berry Bites with Antioxidants

Description: For chocolate fans, this delicious, antioxidant-rich energy bite with dark chocolate, mixed berries, and almonds is a guilt-free pleasure.

Size of Serving: 10 Bits

20 minutes for preparation

Ingredients:

- ½ cup of mixed berries, including raspberries, blueberries, and strawberries
- one-half cup almonds
- 1/4 cup chips made with dark chocolate
- Double-stick of almond butter
- One spoonful of honey

Preparation Guide:

1. Process the mixed berries, almonds, dark chocolate chips, almond butter, and honey in a food processor until thoroughly incorporated.
2. Before serving, roll the mixture into bite-sized balls and place in the refrigerator for at least 30 minutes.

Nutrient-dense ingredients are combined with delicious flavors and textures in these superfood energy bite recipes. These bite-sized snacks are a handy and nutritious way to satisfy your cravings for the crunch of nuts or the sweetness of dried fruits when you need a fast energy boost. Savor the healthy deliciousness of these mouthwatering energy snacks!

Nutrient-Rich Trail Mixes

<u>Trail Mix for Tropical Paradise</u>

Description: Nutrient-rich and invigorating, this tropical combination of nuts, coconut, and dried **fruits is perfect for on-the-go adventures.**

Serving size: 1/4 cup

Five minutes to prepare

Ingredients:

- one-half cup almonds
- Half a cup of dried pineapple pieces
- quarter cup cashews
- 1/4 cup of coconut, shredded

Preparation Guide:

1. In a dish, mix together almonds, cashews, dried pineapple, and shredded coconut.
2. Blend well and divide into 1/4 cup halves.

Enormous Crunch Blend

Description: A crunchy, nutrient-rich trail mix with a hint of dark chocolate, mixed seeds, and almonds makes for a filling and healthful snack.

Serving size: 1/4 cup

Five minutes to prepare

Ingredients:

- one-fourth cup pumpkin seeds
- one-fourth cup sunflower seeds
- Almonds, 1/4 cup
- two tsp worth of dark chocolate chips

Preparation Guide:

1. In a dish, mix together almonds, dark chocolate chips, sunflower seeds, and pumpkin seeds.
2. Blend well and divide into 1/4 cup halves.

Berry Nut Medley Mix

Description: A tasty and nourishing trail mix made with a wonderful blend of nuts and dried berries that is naturally sweet and full of antioxidants.

Serving size: 1/4 cup

Five minutes to prepare

Ingredients:

- Quarter cup walnuts

* 1/4 cup of cranberries, dried
* Pistachios, 1/4 cup
* Almonds, 1/4 cup

Preparation Guide:

1. In a dish, mix together almonds, pistachios, walnuts, and dried cranberries.
2. Blend well and divide into 1/4 cup halves.

Crunch Mix Mediterranean

Description: Roasted chickpeas, olives, and a combination of nuts combine to create a flavorful, high-protein trail mix with a Mediterranean flair that makes for a filling snack.

Serving size: 1/4 cup

Ten minutes to prepare.

Cooking time for roasted chickpeas is twenty minutes.

Ingredients:

* 1/4 cup of roasted lentils
* Almonds, 1/4 cup
* 1/4 cup of olives, green
* 1/4 cup of crumbled feta cheese

Preparation Guide:

1. Bake the chickpeas until they get crispy.
2. In a bowl, mix together feta cheese, almonds, green olives, and roasted chickpeas.
3. Blend well and divide into 1/4 cup halves.

Hot Trailblazer Blend

Description: A robust and hot trail mix with hints of dried mango, seeds, and almonds flavored with chilies for a tasty and energizing snack.

Serving size: 1/4 cup

Five minutes to prepare

Ingredients:

- ½ cup mixed nuts, including peanuts, cashews, and almonds
- one-fourth cup pumpkin seeds
- 1/4 cup chopped dried mango
- A single tsp of chili powder

Preparation Guide:

1. In a dish, combine the dried mango, pumpkin seeds, mixed nuts, and chili powder.
2. Blend well and divide into 1/4 cup halves.

Trail Mix for Chocolate Lovers

Description: For those who love chocolate, this rich trail mix of cashews, goji berries, and dark chocolate-covered almonds is a delicious and nutrient-dense treat.

Serving size: 1/4 cup

Five minutes to prepare

Ingredients:

- 1/4 cup almonds coated in dark chocolate
- Goji berries, 1/4 cup
- quarter cup cashews

Preparation Guide:

1. Put cashews, goji berries, and almonds wrapped in dark chocolate in a dish.
2. Blend well and divide into 1/4 cup halves.

Harvest Mix of Cinnamon and Apples

Description: A trail mix with an autumn theme that includes nuts, dried apple pieces, and almonds seasoned with cinnamon for a hearty and satisfying snack.

Serving size: 1/4 cup

Five minutes to prepare

Ingredients:

- 1/4 cup almonds seasoned with cinnamon
- Slices of dried apple, 1/4 cup
- Pecans, 1/4 cup

Preparation Guide:

1. Put nuts, dried apple pieces, and almonds seasoned with cinnamon in a bowl.
2. Blend well and divide into 1/4 cup halves.

Trail Mix Trailblazer

Description: A filling and nutritious trail mix that combines nuts, seeds, and dried fruits to make a satisfying and well-balanced snack for outdoor activities.

Serving size: 1/4 cup

Five minutes to prepare

Ingredients:

- one-fourth cup sunflower seeds
- Almonds, 1/4 cup
- 1/4 cup chopped dried apricots
- one-fourth cup pumpkin seeds

Preparation Guide:

1. In a dish, mix together sunflower seeds, almonds, dried apricots, and pumpkin seeds.
2. Blend well and divide into 1/4 cup halves.

Spice Mix with Ginger and Turmeric

A tasty and health-promoting snack, this trail mix contains cashews, dried mango, and crystallized ginger along with the anti-inflammatory properties of turmeric and ginger.

Serving size: 1/4 cup

Five minutes to prepare

Ingredients:

- quarter cup cashews

- 1/4 cup chopped dried mango
- 1/2 tsp powdered turmeric
- 1/4 cup minced crystallized ginger

Preparation Guide:

1. In a bowl, combine cashews, powdered turmeric, dried mango, and crystallized ginger.
2. Blend well and divide into 1/4 cup halves.

Crunch Mix with Sesame Honey

Description: A tasty and wholesome trail mix that combines dried blueberries, sesame sticks, and honey-roasted almonds for a wonderful and filling snack.

Serving size: 1/4 cup

Five minutes to prepare

Cooking time for honey-roasted almonds is ten minutes.

Ingredients:

- 1/4 cup almonds toasted with honey
- 1/4 cup of sticks sesame
- 1/4 cup of blueberries, dry

Preparation Guide:

- Almonds should be roasted with honey until golden, then cooled.
- In a bowl, mix sesame sticks, honey-roasted almonds, and dried blueberries.
- Blend well and divide into 1/4 cup halves.

With a range of tastes and textures, these nutrient-dense trail mix recipes provide a satisfying and healthful snack at any time of day. Whether you like your trail mixes with a fiery kick, a chocolaty delight, or a tropical twist, these combinations will fulfill your appetites and provide your body with vital nutrients. Savor the deliciousness of these handmade mixes!

Sweet and Savory Superfood Snack Recipes

Parmesan-Crusted Kale Chips

Description: A tasty and nutrient-rich substitute for typical snacks, crispy kale chips are seasoned with Parmesan cheese.

Serving Size: Two

10-minute prep

Preparation Time: 15 minutes

Ingredients:

- One bundle of dried and cleaned kale
- Two tsp of olive oil
- 1/4 cup of Parmesan cheese, grated
- Add pepper and salt to taste.

Preparation Guide:

1. Set oven temperature to 175°C/350°F.

2. Take off the kale leaves' stems and shred them into little pieces.
3. Combine the kale, olive oil, Parmesan, salt, and pepper in a bowl.
4. Place on a baking sheet, then bake until crispy, about 15 minutes.

Almond-Blueberry Energy Bites

Description: Blueberries, almonds, and oats come together in these no-bake energy bites to create a delightful and filling snack.

Size of Serving: 10 Bits

15 minutes for preparation

Ingredients:

- 1 cup of blueberries, dry
- cup of almonds
- Oats, rolled, one cup
- halved cup honey

Preparation Guide:

1. Blend the oats, almonds, and blueberries in a food processor.
2. Blend the items until they are well-chopped.
3. After adding the honey, pulse the ingredients to create a sticky dough.
4. Shape into little balls and keep chilled for a minimum of 60 minutes.

Trail Mix with Quinoa and Cranberries

Description: A high-protein trail mix that is ideal for on-the-go eating, including quinoa, almonds, and cranberries.

Cup of serving size

Five minutes to prepare

Preparation Time: 15 minutes

Ingredients:

- Half a cup of chilled, cooked quinoa
- Almonds, 1/4 cup
- 1/4 cup of cranberries, dried
- One spoonful of honey

Preparation Guide:

1. Combine the quinoa, almonds, and cranberries in a dish.
2. Over the mixture, drizzle with honey and toss until thoroughly mixed.
3. Arrange onto a baking sheet and bake, stirring regularly, at 350°F (175°C) for 15 minutes.

Bruschetta with Avocado and Tomato

Description: A delicious whole-grain bread bruschetta with avocado, cherry tomatoes, and basil.

Serving size: 4 slices

Ten minutes to prepare.

Five minutes for cooking

Ingredients:

- 1 chopped avocado
- Half a cup of cherry tomatoes
- Four pieces of whole-grain bread, toasted with freshly chopped basil

Preparation Guide:

1. Combine chopped basil, cherry tomatoes, and cubed avocado in a bowl.
2. Transfer the mixture onto pieces of toasted wholegrain bread.

<u>Roasted Chickpeas with Turmeric</u>

Description: Crunchy and tasty snack with anti-inflammatory properties made from roasted chickpeas seasoned with cumin and turmeric.

Cup of serving size

Ten minutes to prepare.

Cooking Period: Half an hour

Ingredients:

- One can (15 oz) of rinsed and drained chickpeas
- One tsp of olive oil
- One tsp of turmeric
- One-half tsp cumin
- Add salt to taste.

Preparation Guide:

1. Turn the oven on to 400°F, or 200°C.
2. Gently pat dry chickpeas with a paper towel.
3. Combine chickpeas, cumin, turmeric, and olive oil in a bowl.
4. Place on a baking sheet, then bake until crispy, about 30 minutes.

Black bean and sweet potato salsa

Description: This salsa, which pairs well with whole-grain tortilla chips, is a delightful blend of sweet potatoes, black beans, corn, and cilantro.

Size: Two Cups

15 minutes for preparation

Preparation Time: 20 minutes

Ingredients:

- One big sweet potato, chopped
- One can (15 oz) of rinsed and drained black beans
- One cup of kernel corn
- chopped fresh cilantro

Preparation Guide:

- Sweet potatoes should be roasted or steam-cooked until soft.
- Sweet potatoes, black beans, corn, and cilantro should all be combined in a dish.

Edamame with Mango and Chili

Description: Mango, chili-lime flavor, sea salt, and spicy edamame with a touch of the tropics.

Cup of serving size

Five minutes to prepare

Five minutes for cooking

Ingredients:

- One cup of steamed edamame
- 1/2 cup of mango dice
- Lime and chili seasoning
- to taste sea salt

Preparation Guide:

1. Combine chopped mango and steamed edamame in a bowl.
2. Season with the chile lime and sea salt.

Quinoa Bars with Almonds and Dark Chocolate

Description: Wholesome and filling quinoa bars loaded with nutrients, paired with dark chocolate and almonds.

Size of Serving: 8 bars

15 minutes for preparation

Preparation Time: 25 minutes

Ingredients:

- 1 cup of quinoa, cooked
- Half a cup of chopped almonds
- 1/4 cup chips made with dark chocolate
- 1/4 cup of honey.

Preparation Guide:

1. Set oven temperature to 175°C/350°F.
2. Combine the quinoa, honey, dark chocolate chips, and chopped almonds in a bowl.
3. Transfer the blend onto a baking dish and cook it for twenty-five minutes.

Hummus and Cucumber Bites

Description: A simple and nutritious snack of crisp cucumber slices garnished with cherry tomatoes, hummus, and black sesame seeds.

Size of Serving: 2

Ten minutes to prepare.

Cooking Period: Not at all

Ingredients:

- 1 sliced cucumber with hummus
- Half a cherry tomato
- Sesame seeds, black, to garnish

Preparation Guide:

1. Place slices of cucumber on a serving dish.

2. Place a cherry tomato half and a dollop of hummus on top
   of each cucumber slice.
3. Add black sesame seeds as a garnish.

Energy Balls with Coconut and Matcha

Description: Flavorful and stimulating snack, coconut, matcha,
and almond butter come together in these no-bake energy balls.

Balls in serving size: ten

15 minutes for preparation

Ingredients:

- One cup of coconut shreds
- Twice as much matcha powder
- 50 ml of almond butter
- 1/4 cup of honey.

Preparation Guide:

1. Combine the shredded coconut, almond butter, honey, and
   matcha powder in a bowl.
2. Refrigerate the mixture for at least an hour after rolling it
   into bite-sized balls.

These recipes for savory and sweet superfood snacks offer a range
of tastes and textures, satisfying cravings while also offering health
advantages. These dishes, which include a crispy chip substitute, a
trail mix full of protein, or a delicious bruschetta, are made with
healthy ingredients to make snacking more enjoyable. Savor these
tasty and wholesome treats!

Chapter 6

Meal Planning for Lifelong Wellness

Your diet has a major role in determining your level of wellbeing throughout your life. Meal planning is an essential tactic for fueling your body, promoting general health, and creating the groundwork for a fulfilling life. It is not only a weight-management technique.

The Basis for Wellbeing

The foundation of a comprehensive approach to wellbeing is meal planning. It serves as a proactive approach to fulfill nutritional demands, fuel energy, and increase lifespan, going beyond simple feeding. Planning your meals with intention gives you the power to make decisions that support your body's needs and promote long-term health.

Essential Guidelines for Efficient Meal Planning

1. Balanced Nutrition: A diverse diet plan welcomes a range of foods. Incorporate a variety of nutrient-dense meals, including whole grains, lean meats, vibrant veggies, and healthy fats. To make sure you satisfy your body's diverse nutritional demands, aim for balance.

2. Mindful Portioning: It's critical to comprehend portion amounts. Portion control helps avoid consuming too much of some nutrients and also helps with weight management. You can appreciate tastes and respect your body's cues of hunger and fullness by controlling your portion sizes.

3. Adventure and Variety: Celebrate the diversity of cuisines. Eating a diversified diet exposes your body to a wide range of nutrients and enhances the enjoyment of meals. To keep your palate interested, try a variety of dishes, ingredients, and cooking techniques.

4. Integration of Hydration: Water is an essential component of wellbeing that is sometimes disregarded. Include meals and drinks high in water in your meal plan. Drinking enough water, herbal teas, or hydrating fruits may all help you keep properly hydrated, which is very beneficial to your general health.

5. Sustainable Practices: Think about how your food choices affect the health of the earth and yourself. Selecting foods that are ethically and sustainably sourced will benefit both the environment and your health.

The Advantages of Careful Meal Planning

1. Optimized Nutrition: By organizing your meals, you may customize your diet to fit your unique nutritional needs. A carefully planned meal plan serves as a road map for accomplishing your objectives, whether they be maintaining energy levels, increasing immunity, or promoting heart health and wellness.

2. Efficiency of Time and Resources: Meal preparation ahead of time conserves both. It simplifies grocery shopping, lessens food waste, and removes the need for last-minute selections. This effectiveness encourages a steady and long-term attitude to eating healthily.

3. Empowerment in Decisions: Taking charge of your meal preparation gives you the ability to choose what you eat with awareness and knowledge. It encourages a healthy relationship with food, viewing each meal as a chance to fuel your body and advance your overall wellbeing for the rest of your life.

4. Weight Management and Beyond: Meal planning has several advantages that go far beyond the scale when it comes to managing weight. It has a good impact on mood, vitality, mental clarity, and the body's ability to withstand a range of health difficulties.

Useful Advice for Effective Meal Planning

1. Make sensible objectives:

Start with attainable goals. Modest adjustments have a higher chance of becoming ingrained behaviors. When defining your objectives, take into account your interests, way of life, and any dietary constraints.

2. Batch Cooking and Preparation:

Prepare meal components ahead of time to save time during the week. On hectic days, batch cooking grains, proteins, and cutting veggies may save time and increase accessibility to nutritious options.

3. Adaptability and Flexibility: Because life is unpredictable, your diet plan should be adaptable. Accept flexibility and make necessary alterations in response to day-to-day needs.

4. Attentive Eating Practices: Practice being attentive while you eat. Chew gently, appreciate tastes, and pay attention to your body's signals of hunger and fullness. Eating mindfully improves the whole nutrition experience.

Meal planning is essentially a dynamic and powerful activity that promotes lifetime fitness. It's a dedication to respecting your body by making deliberate, health-conscious decisions. Through putting nutrition first, accepting diversity, and implementing sustainable habits, you set out on a path that leads to a lifetime of wellbeing rather than simply a nutritious meal.

Tailoring Superfoods to Individual Health Goals

One size does not fit all when it comes to achieving optimal health. Customizing superfoods to meet specific requirements has become a fundamental component of personalized nutrition, since it acknowledges the distinctive and ever-changing character of each person's health objectives. This sophisticated method accounts for each person's unique nutritional needs as well as their overall health goals, such as weight loss, heightened energy, or specific wellbeing.

Accepting Individualization in Diet

Comprehending Personal Health Objectives

Everybody sets out on a health journey with different goals in mind. Some may desire to get rid of extra weight, while others may want to gain muscle or improve their mental acuity. Customizing superfoods to meet personal health goals requires a deep comprehension of these targets in order to make sure that dietary decisions support the intended results.

Adapting Nutrition Profiles

Superfoods, which are renowned for having high concentrations of vital nutrients, can be effective allies when tailored to meet specific health needs. The selection of superfoods may be precisely calibrated to provide a customized nutritional profile that supports specific health objectives, whether one desires antioxidants for skin health, omega-3 fatty acids for heart wellness, or protein for muscular building.

Getting Around the Superfood Landscape for Weight Loss and Metabolic Health

Superfoods like chia seeds, kale, and green tea can be essential for achieving weight management and better metabolic health. These components help the body achieve a healthy weight by improving metabolic efficiency in addition to providing satiety.

Sports Efficiency and Muscle Growth

Superfoods high in protein, such quinoa, lentils, and spirulina, are beneficial for those who are involved in exercise and muscle growth. These nutrient-dense foods support physical activity, facilitate muscle repair, and increase the body's general strength and resilience.

Mental Acuity and Mental Clarity

Superfoods such as fatty salmon, walnuts, and blueberries are important for cognitive wellness. Their omega-3 fatty acids and neuroprotective qualities are well known for boosting mental clarity, improving focus, and maintaining brain health.

Creating Customized Superfood Plans and Consulting Nutrition Specialists

Achieving individualized nutrition frequently entails working with nutrition specialists who can identify unique health requirements and create customized superfood regimens. These experts consider variables like age, gender, degree of exercise, and pre-existing medical issues to make sure the superfoods they choose complement each person's objectives.

Changing Health Dynamics: Adapting

Personal health objectives are dynamic; they change over time and in response to new situations. One of the most important aspects of customizing superfoods to meet personal demands is flexibility.

Frequent evaluations in conjunction with modifications to the superfood repertory guarantee that nutrition stays in balance with the fluctuations of personal health dynamics.

A customized strategy for well-being

Customization is the key to obtaining the full range of health advantages when it comes to superfoods. By customizing superfoods to meet each person's unique health objectives, we empower people on their wellness journeys and provide the foundation for a healthy and sustainable lifestyle. Personalized nutrition in conjunction with the natural power of superfoods represents a paradigm leap in health care, making each person's path to transformational well-being as distinct as they are.

Weekly Meal Planning Guide

Set Your Objectives: First things first, decide what your dietary objectives are: weight loss, muscle gain, more energy, or general health.

Daily Meal Schedule:

<u>Monday: Get Things Going:</u>

Breakfast consists of a nutrient-dense smoothie bowl topped with Greek yogurt and mixed berries.

Lunch would be a lean protein source, such as tofu or grilled chicken, along with a quinoa salad and roasted veggies.

Dinner is steamed broccoli and baked fish with sweet potatoes.

Tuesday: Power of Proteins:

Whole grain toast and spinach-and-egg scrambles are the **breakfas**t staples.

Lunch would be whole-grain crackers and mixed greens served alongside lentil soup.

Supper is bell peppers filled with quinoa and green beans on the side.

Wednesday: A Pleasure with Plants:

Avocado toast for **breakfast**, topped with chia seeds and cherry tomatoes.

Brown rice stir-fried with vegetables and chickpeas for **lunch.**

Dinner is grilled shrimp served with zucchini noodles and tomato sauce.

Thursday: Focus on Hydration:

Breakfast consists of chia seeds, almond milk, and fresh fruit mixed with overnight oats.

Lunch is refreshing wraps made with cucumbers and hummus with a side of watermelon.

Dinner is a beautiful salad of grilled chicken with a variety of veggies.

Friday: Moderate Indulgence

Greek yogurt topped with mixed berries and whole-grain pancakes for **breakfast**.

Lunch is a quinoa dish dressed with cilantro, lime, and black beans, as well as corn and avocado.

Supper is brown rice and broccoli with stir-fried tofu.

Saturday: Day of Recuperation:

Smoothie with bananas and almond butter for **breakfast.**

Lunch is an omelette with spinach and feta served with whole-grain bread.

Supper is baked cod over quinoa and asparagus.

Sunday: Prepare dinner and unwind:

Greek yogurt parfait with fresh fruit and oats for **breakfast**.

Lunch consists of prepared quinoa and grilled veggie bowls.

Supper is plant-based protein or lean ground turkey over a slow cooker with chili.

Advice and Methods:

Combined Cooking: To make meal preparation during the week easier, prepare huge quantities of basics like quinoa, roasted veggies, and lean meats.

Snack Wisely: To maintain consistent energy levels in between meals, include wholesome snacks like fresh fruit, mixed nuts, and chopped vegetables with hummus.

Remain Hydrated: Make drinking water a priority throughout the day. For some variation, try adding herbal teas or infused water.

The key is flexibility: Give yourself leeway while creating your food plan. Maintain a balanced diet while making adjustments for unforeseen circumstances, social commitments, and desires.

Creating a weekly meal plan is an active step in reaching your dietary objectives. This plan acts as a roadmap, giving a varied and well-balanced selection of meals along with the adaptability required to adjust to the ever-changing circumstances of everyday living. A great weekly meal plan is built on consistency, diversity, and thoughtful selections. This creates a wholesome and sustainable strategy to fuelling your week with purpose.

Adapting Superfoods for Different Lifestyles (e.g., busy professionals, families, fitness enthusiasts)

First of all,

Recognizing Different Lifestyles

Acknowledge the distinct needs and inclinations of many lifestyles, including the hectic schedules of professionals, the ever-changing requirements of families, and the fitness-focused regimens of enthusiasts.

Lifestyle-Based Superfood Remedies:

Intentional Professionals:

Mobile Nutrition:

Offer nutrient-dense energy snacks, trail mix with nuts and dried fruits, and chia seed pudding as portable superfood alternatives.

Provide easy smoothie recipes that may be made ahead of time and enjoyed during busy workdays.

Snacks Perfect for a Desk:

Suggest nutritious and easy lunchtime snacks that are desk-friendly, such as individual pieces of Greek yogurt with honey, mixed almonds, and kale chips.

Quick and Easy Meal Planning:

Stress the value of prepping adaptable superfood foundation, like quinoa and roasted veggies, for easy, fast meals that can be customized.

For households:

Superfoods Suitable for Kids:

Blend veggies into spaghetti sauces, add chia seeds to yogurt, and gently add spinach to smoothies to introduce superfoods into family favorites.

Make interactive food stations so kids may examine cut-up fruits, vegetables, and dips.

Family Bonding Over Meals:

Stress the value of family dinners and get the family involved in choosing the superfoods for the weekly menus.

Share kid-friendly dishes with them, such as bright salads, homemade granola bars, or tacos packed with superfoods.

Easy Superfood Substitutes:

Provide simple substitutions for common ingredients in family recipes, such as whole-grain flour, sweet potatoes, or lean meats like tofu or fish.

For Those Who Love Fitness:

Pre-Exertion Fuel

For a pre-workout boost, suggest superfoods like oats, bananas, and almonds that offer prolonged energy.

Draw attention to how important it is to stay hydrated by adding superfood ingredients, such as cucumber or berries, to your water.

After-Work out Healing:

Provide advice on high-protein superfoods for efficient post-workout recuperation, such as Greek yogurt, chia seeds, and lean meats.

To refuel, promote nutrient-dense smoothies made with fruits, protein powder, and spinach.

Timing and composition of meals:

A manual on the best times and types of meals, with a focus on the significance of a well-balanced combination of healthy fats, proteins, and carbs.

For accelerated healing, promote the use of superfoods that reduce inflammation, such as ginger and turmeric.

All-purpose Advice on Flexibility:

Being adaptable when preparing:

Offer flexible recipes that accommodate varying cooking styles, such as rapid stir-fries, one-pan bakes, or large-scale meals prepared in bulk.

Replace Superfoods:

Provide superfood substitutes for everyday foods to facilitate a smooth assimilation into daily activities.

Teaching Materials:

Provide enlightening materials such as leaflets or web content to enable people to make decisions based on their lifestyles.

Customizing superfoods to fit various lifestyles requires careful planning. People may easily include these nutrient-dense solutions into their everyday life by customizing recommendations to meet the specific needs of families, fitness enthusiasts, and busy professionals. Regardless of their varied and dynamic schedules, everyone may make the transition to a healthy lifestyle pleasurable and attainable with the help of easily accessible solutions.

Conclusion

Now that we've reached the last chapter of the "Real Superfoods Diet Cookbook," I want to sincerely thank you for coming along on this gastronomic journey to long-term health. Our trip through more than 120 delicious and healthful meals has been nothing short of remarkable, and I hope it has permanently changed the way you think about fueling yourself naturally.

We haven't just discussed recipes in these pages; we've developed a way of life—a celebration of healthful, nutrient-dense, and delicious meals that are in sync with your body, mind, and spirit. Our collaborative culinary canvas serves as evidence that eating for wellness can be an artistic endeavor, a way to express one's love for oneself, and a voyage of exploration.

A Harmony of Tastes and Elements

These chapters' recipes are carefully designed to balance tastes, textures, and nutritional value. Every meal is a harmony of health on your plate, from the vivid colors of nutrient-dense fruits and vegetables to the cozy warmth of filling grains and proteins.

Beyond the Plate: A Change in Way of Life

However, this cookbook is a catalyst for a change in lifestyle rather than just a list of dishes. It's an encouragement to see food as a powerful source of energy, life, and happiness, rather than just something to eat. It's a manual for adopting a true superfoods diet that goes beyond diet trends and is a lasting and fulfilling way of living.

Taking Charge of Your Wellness Journey

I hope the lessons stick with you and the tastes linger as you appreciate the last pages. May this cookbook encourage you to make thoughtful decisions, stimulate your creativity in the kitchen, and give you self-assurance that you can put your health first.

Your Well-Being, Your Jewel

Recall that every meal is a brushstroke in the painting that is your wellness journey. You feed not just your body with each food, but also your dreams of living a long, healthy, and happy life.

A Heartfelt Goodbye

As we say goodbye to our culinary journey, I urge you to incorporate the spirit of these dishes into your everyday routine. Allow the genuine superfoods diet's tenets to serve as a compass for you as you move toward a lifetime of wellbeing.

I appreciate you sharing a little portion of your wellness journey with me. May you always see your kitchen as a painting for robust health and may every meal be an occasion to celebrate the incredible trip that is your life.

To your well-being, joy, and an abundance of delectable and fulfilling times ahead.

THANK YOU